The Health of Your Dog

The
Health of Your Dog

John Bower & David Youngs

The Crowood Press

First published in 1989 by
The Crowood Press
Gipsy Lane, Swindon
Wiltshire SN2 6DQ

Reprinted 1990

British Library Cataloguing in Publication Data

Bower, John
   The health of your dog.
   1. Livestock: Dogs. Veterinary aspects
   I. Title II. Youngs, David
   636.7'089

   ISBN 1–85223–145–9

To Boony and Becky, Sophie and Rachel
To Jennie, Jane and Rachel

Line-Drawings by Aileen Hanson

Typeset by Columns of Reading
Printed in Great Britain by Butler & Tanner Ltd, Frome and London

'Why don't you become a vet?'

Patrick De Ville. November, 1959.

'Now you are qualified, I'll teach you how to treat clients.'

Frank W. Beattie. September, 1965.

'A veterinary surgeon's role is to heal animals; dog collars and grooming brushes have no place in the waiting room.'

W. Brian Singleton. April, 1988.

Contents

Foreword

We all care for our dogs, but caring is not enough. Caring without knowing means that we are often bewildered in the face of illness and accidents.

Knowing about animals is fascinating for the animal lover, and to the responsible dog owner who is eager to widen his knowledge this book is a treasure house. It is not simply a book of casual hints and tips, it is a comprehensive manual of information dealing exhaustively with every ailment and contingency likely to be encountered.

It is a known fact that people often worry more about their dogs' troubles than they do about their own. As a practising vet myself I know this to be true and as a dedicated dog owner I understand their feeling of helplessness when they are confronted with symptoms and behaviour which they do not understand. How comforting then to be able to turn to this book and find an explanation of the things that are causing their anxiety. It is all there, easy to find and presented in simple language.

It is not meant to take the place of a veterinary surgeon, but it can alert the owner to the need to seek professional advice and, when his pet is under veterinary care, it can help the owner to see beneath the surface and to follow the course of treatment with insight and comprehension. This helps everybody – especially the dog.

The desire to understand a pet animal is a very deep and fundamental one, and when it is realised it results in a closer and more secure relationship. One wants to help not only when a dog is ill but when he behaves in an unusual way. Behavioural problems are a growing and vastly interesting field in veterinary work and one which is being explored more and more deeply. When I look back over the idiosyncrasies of the many dogs I have had I realise more and more than the canine race is almost as susceptible to psychological peculiarities as the human one. Some of these things can be funny but others deeply worrying and the book contains valuable information on this. And it is good to be able to recognise and be forearmed against the difficulties which can arise during normal processes, such as breeding and whelping.

Greatly helpful, too, are the chapters on the care of the healthy dog, the recognition of the signs of good health, correct diet and the choice of a suitable puppy. We are taken by the hand and led through the dog's life, discussing on the way the widely varying problems which arise from puppyhood to old age.

The authors are vastly experienced men dealing daily with the countless ailments, mental and physical, of dogs in their veterinary hospital. Their findings and their words of advice are based not on theoretical notions or ideas but on personally proven facts. Their book is not only a superb volume of reference; just browsing through it is a rewarding experience, and a thorough perusal of its pages will be an exciting voyage of discovery for any dog lover.

James Herriot

Acknowledgements

Our thanks go to all those who have helped us during the development of this book, expecially our partner, Philip Hunt, for his tolerance of our use of practice personnel and facilities, and our colleagues, who with patience have helped us select cases for photographs. We would like to thank Dr Roger Mugford for his help with the chapter on behavioural problems, and Jacqui Jones and Joan Simmons who read much of the material and provided helpful comments. Thanks are also due to our clients who allowed us to photograph them and their dogs. We are especially grateful to Nigel Rolstone for providing most of the black and white photographs and to Marc Henrie for his skill in obtaining the cover photograph. Other photographs were generously supplied by Dr Peter Bedford, Dr John Houlton, Dr Keith Thoday and the late Dr Charlie Mackenzie, Sophie Bower, Ray Butcher, Roger Williams, Zena Andrews, Marc Henrie ASC for the cover photograph of Dot, Glen and John, Frank Garwood and Pedigree Petfoods. But our particular thanks are due to Jennie Youngs who patiently translated our writings into English, Caroline Bower for monitoring our accuracy, and above all to Caroline Price our practice secretary who typed, retyped and typed again the entire manuscript.

Introduction

In recent years, the increasing importance of the pet dog within the family and a greater interest in dog showing and breeding, has led to a more widespread awareness of, and desire for, knowledge of the dog's health status. It is fair to say that the dog is regarded by most owners (ourselves included) as one of the family, and his health and illnesses are of great concern to us. When he is ill, we want to know the nature of the problem, how it is treated and how it can be avoided in the future. This book is aimed at the responsible dog owner who wishes to learn more about the dog and his special disease problems, but is written in a more readable form than the usual reference books. Because the dog is one of the family, we have not used the pronoun 'it' in the book, but rather have referred to the dog as 'he' or 'she'. Where our comments apply equally to male or female we have used 'he' to avoid the messy 'he/she' combination and we hope owners of bitches will forgive us. Where the problem is specific to a bitch we have of course referred to her as 'she'.

This owners' veterinary manual begins with the dog in his healthy state and gives guide-lines on how to recognise if he is indeed healthy. This section also explains the pack behaviour which is normal to all dogs, from wild wolves and foxes to pet Golden Retrievers, and consequently how the domesticated dog views his place in his family or pack. It explains the all-important development of the relationship with the puppy as he grows to adulthood and the consequent avoidance of many future be-havioural problems. The sources of new puppies or adult dogs are listed, with recommendations, and the section on how to choose the correct puppy for one's life-style should prevent mistakes being made. Management, care and feeding of the new arrival are comprehensively covered.

During the growth phase of the puppy, certain special disease problems occur. These are explained and practical suggestions put forward on how to avoid them. A chapter on the common infectious diseases of the dog follows, complete with symptoms, treatment that the vet and the owner can give, and methods of prevention.

The bulk of the manual examines the dog system by system, firstly describing the normal structure and function of each system, and then the more common disease problems, with their symptoms and treatment. Useful chapters then follow on breeding and associated problems, behavioural problems with their correction and prevention, and first aid, accidents and emergencies. The final chapter deals with the special problems of the older dog and includes a section on the emotive subject of euthanasia.

This book is written in practical, easily understood terms and deals with the common problems as seen in a busy, small animal Veterinary Hospital practice employing seven vets. It is not intended as a replacement for the veterinary surgeon or the more usual A–Z dictionary of diseases, but it is hoped it will become a readable reference book for the interested dog owner.

1 The Healthy Dog

To understand your dog and how he behaves as part of your family, it is necessary to consider both the instinctive behaviour of his ancestors and wild counterparts, and his adaptation to living with man for centuries.

ORIGINS

The original domesticated dogs are thought to have been camp followers at a time when man was nomadic and lived in small tribes. These wild dogs who cleared food debris from the campsite were gradually welcomed into the camp for this purpose. They also provided warmth and security for the humans. Gradually, their use and acceptance widened until today most pet dogs are regarded as one of the family.

PACK BEHAVIOUR

The wolf is a near relative of the domestic dog, and his pack behaviour gives us an insight into how to regard and react to the dog within our family, his pack. Within the wolf pack there is a definite social structure, with a pack leader and a pecking order of subordinates. The pack leader will, of course, be challenged from time to time by maturing male wolves but he will retain his position by demonstrating his authority through posture, behaviour and voice. Only rarely will serious fighting occur. He is the strongest, most intelligent wolf in the pack and this ensures the survival of the pack. Eventually, he will be replaced by a stronger rival. Within the pack there is a pecking order so that each wolf, or group of wolves, knows his place. Much more fighting occurs at the middle levels of the hierarchy than at the top. The weak do not challenge and, therefore, they come to no harm.

So it is with the domestic dog. The owner must be the leader of the pack, whether the pack is just one owner and dog, or a whole family and dog. For a successful and happy relationship, it is essential that the dog is the subordinate member of the whole family. This position is usually easy to achieve and, once settled and reinforced from time to time, the dog is an extremely happy, secure and obedient member of the family. It is not sufficient for one member, say the husband, to be the pack leader as this can lead to problems when the dog is disciplined or given a command by another member of the family. In such a situation, children are usually at the bottom of the pecking order, but whoever it is may suffer bites and aggression. Sadly, this type of problem is commonly presented at the surgery, but it can usually be prevented by establishing dominance immediately the dog becomes a member of the family. Chapter 17, on behavioural problems, covers this and many other problems that need to be considered in the light of pack behaviour. The two-way relationship thus established remains a pleasure for the whole family, including the dog, for life.

RELATIONSHIP WITH MAN

The relationship that develops between people and their dogs is very strong indeed.

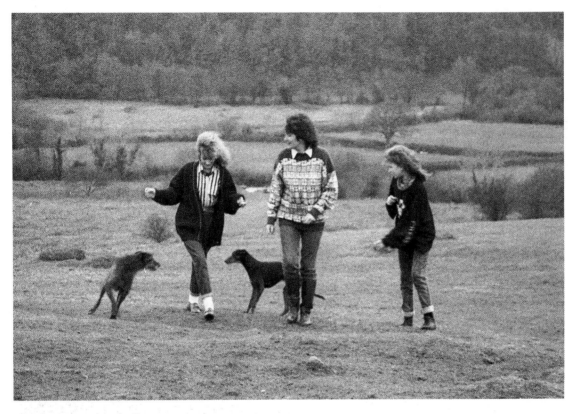

Your dog as part of the family.

Until one has owned a dog, it is difficult to realise how important the dog is within the family unit. Research shows that, nowadays, the dog is regarded as a member of the family, equivalent to a child of between three to ten years (not a child substitute, or surrogate, but an equivalent member). We talk to the dog, play games with him, discipline him, feed him, spoil him and chastise him using the same level of conversation that we would with a child of that age. Furthermore, when we lose the dog, whether unexpectedly or with age, we suffer enormous grief. The relationship is powerful and two-way; the dog derives as much pleasure and security out of it as the owner. He is, without question, faithful and loving and makes no judgement on his owner.

This characteristic has led to the dog's successful involvement in certain forms of medical therapy. Mentally ill patients or long-term prisoners can often communicate with dogs but may not be able to relate to humans. Pet dogs are marvellous therapy for the elderly and lonely, and the dog in the nursing or residential home is an eagerly anticipated visitor. This has been formalised to some extent by the organisation PRO-dogs, whose PAT-dogs (PRO-dog Active Therapy dogs) are taken by their owners to visit people who are lonely or in residential homes. There are currently 4,000 dogs on the PRO-dogs register. In the USA, similar human/companion animal bond organisations exist. The Delta Society, based in Renton, Washington, provides help and advice for all their activities, and

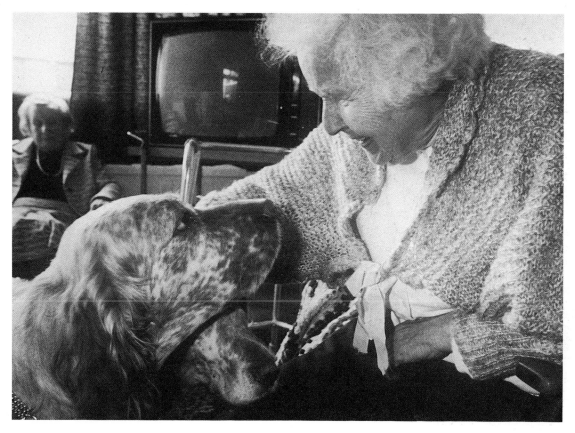

English Setter PAT – dogs visiting.

is the equivalent of the Society for Companion Animal Studies in Great Britain (SCAS).

The human–dog relationship is also responsible for the success of dogs as guide dogs for the blind, hearing dogs for the deaf, sheep dogs and police dogs. There are many other examples where dogs are delighted to be working in the company of humans.

The various breeds of dog have taken a long time to evolve and most were developed for a particular function. Therefore, the breed of dog governs his behaviour, his adaptability and his life style. A hyperactive little Jack Russell Terrier would make a very poor sheep dog or guide dog but he is an excellent rabbiter! A sleepy Bloodhound may not be the best candidate for a hearing dog for the deaf – it would never occur to him to wake up just because the telephone was ringing! Equally, the choice of the correct breed for a family is very important if maximum enjoyment is to be achieved for both the owners and the pet. The time to consider this is before buying the puppy.

HEALTH SIGNS

It does not take a vet to recognise a healthy dog. Most owners can tell their dog is unwell before their vet can because they are attuned to all the small behaviour patterns and characteristics that their dog shows every day. If these change, then something may be wrong.

17

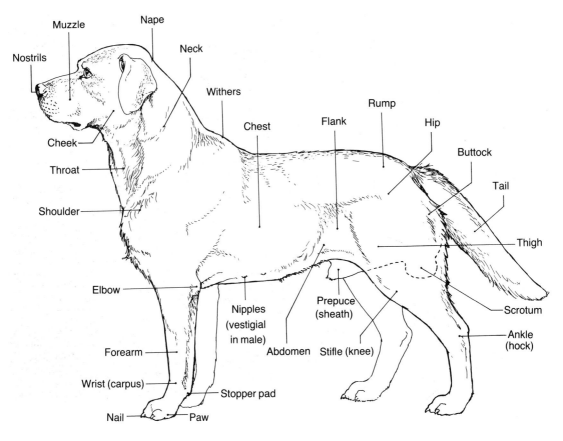

Fig 1 Points of the dog

In general, a healthy dog *looks* healthy. He wants to play with you, as games are a very important part of a dog's life, and he is always ready for his walk.

A healthy dog's eyes are bright and alert. They glisten slightly due to their healthy tear film and, apart from the small amount of sleep in the inner corners, there is no discharge. His nose is usually cold and wet, although a warm nose does not necessarily indicate illness. There should be no discharge from healthy nostrils although a little clear fluid can be normal. His ears are also alert and very responsive to sounds around him, whether it be his food bowl or someone coming up the garden path. The inside of his ear flap is pale pink in appearance and

silky in texture. No wax will be visible and there will be no unpleasant smell. He will only occasionally scratch his ear.

A healthy dog's coat, which you should groom regularly, will be glossy and feel pleasant to the touch. He will not itch excessively and there will be no scurf present. On his skin there will be no bald areas or scabs, and his coat will smell doggy but not unpleasant. He may, however, continuously shed hairs which is referred to as moulting.

The teeth of a healthy dog should be white and smooth. If they are yellow and dull there may be plaque formation, which is a deposit on the teeth formed by chemical change of left-over food particles.

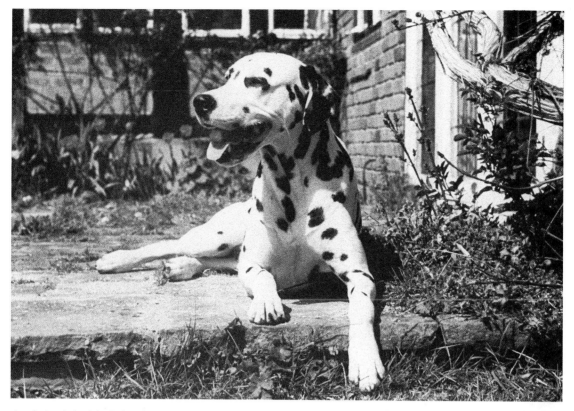

An obviously healthy Dalmatian.

This dental plaque will produce gum disease and there will be inflammation where the tooth meets the gum which will result in a foul smell to his breath (halitosis). The answer, of course, is dentistry which is covered in Chapter 6.

A dog's claws should not be broken or too long. Just like human nails, there is a short non-sensitive tip. The claw should literally end at ground level when the pad is flat on the floor. If it grows too long, the claw will push the toe up and cause pain. However, more often the long claw will break off exposing the sensitive nail bed, which is the equivalent of the pink part of human nails. The front feet always contain four toes, plus a fifth (dew claw) which is equivalent to our thumb. This claw, because it does not touch the ground, will sometimes grow too long and require clipping. Some breeds, such as the Boxer, have these dew claws removed at about three days of age to avoid future problems.

Many breeds are born with just four toes on the hind feet although a number of breeds, and many mongrels, are also born with dew claws. Hind dew claws are more of a problem as they protrude and therefore easily catch on obstacles as the dog bounds about or turns sharply. Again, it is usual for a vet to remove them at about three days of age, although some breeds, such as the Pyrenean Mountain Dog, proudly sport their dew claws which may even be double. These invariably require clipping from time to time. Dogs will not pay much attention to their feet, apart from normal washing, but excessive licking can indicate disease.

A healthy dog will pass stools (faeces) between one and six times a day depending on diet (more roughage, more stools), temperament, breed and opportunity. It is important to realise this normal variation and not worry if the neighbour's dog is very different in his habits. Apart from normal cleaning, a dog will pay little attention to his anus. Excess licking or scooting usually indicates that something is wrong. A male dog will urinate numerous times on a walk as this is territorial behaviour. Bitches, however, urinate less often. An increase in the number of times the dog urinates may indicate disease, especially if accompanied by straining or haemorrhage.

A healthy dog will look in good bodily condition for his size – not too fat and not too thin. Sixty per cent of dogs nowadays are overweight, so be careful not to let your dog join these ranks!

DIET

A dog will usually be ready for his meal and once adult, he should be fed regularly at the same time each day. Most dogs require one meal a day, which should be a balanced meal of protein and carbohydrates plus roughage, vitamins, minerals and trace elements. Some healthy dogs, however, seem to require two meals daily just to maintain a normal weight. These are the very active dogs who tend to burn off more calories.

Most prepared foods provide all the requirements for adult dogs. These foods are available in three forms – moist (canned, cooked and packaged); semi-moist; and dried (biscuit-like consistency). Your vet will be able to tell you which diet is suitable for your dog but only the dog will be able to tell whether he likes it! In general, moist food, such as canned dog food, is highly acceptable to dogs. However,

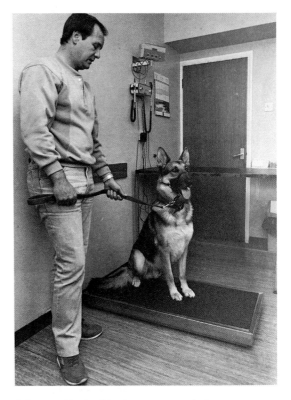

A German Shepherd has his weight checked.

it is important to understand whether the can contains a complete food or one that needs carbohydrate, such as biscuits, mixed in with it. This biscuit provides most of the energy for your dog to use up on exercise so the amount you feed him depends on the level of activity of the dog, and his size. Obesity is caused by feeding more calorie-containing food than is required and these excess calories produce body fat. Thus, on a slimming diet, the calorie intake is restricted and fat deposits are converted back into energy resulting in weight loss. It is important to appreciate that feeding recommendations are only guide-lines. All dogs vary and the important thing is to correlate food with weight and activity.

The biscuit element of the diet also provides roughage, enabling the dog to pass normal stools each day. If his stools are not solid, it may be advisable to increase the roughage by adding some bran or vegetable, such as grated carrot, to his food. Dogs, like humans, need roughage.

Dried prepared food – which is usually cheaper than fresh or canned food – contains adequate amounts of roughage and is a perfectly acceptable diet for dogs, provided attention is paid to water requirements. Of course, a bowl of fresh water should always be available for your dog regardless of his diet.

As you will read in the section on dentistry, a large *raw* marrow bone is a very useful adjunct to a diet as the gnawing process literally cleans the teeth. Hide chew sticks help in this function but they are not as efficient as raw marrow bones. Never be tempted to give your dog cooked bones, sharp chop bones or ribs, as these can cause internal damage.

In our experience, there are two main nutritional problems: obesity and diarrhoea. Both of these problems are usually caused because the owner humanises the dog and feeds the type and quantity of food a human would like to eat. Most dogs do not need much food in comparison with a human. A Miniature Dachshund or a King Charles Spaniel will need only about 250g

(8oz) total food a day, even if he is very lively. 250g (8oz) of food does not look much in a bowl, but it is all he needs. A Labrador may need 700g (1½lb) total food a day or more if he is very active. Never over feed your dog. Conversely, one of the common causes of thin dogs is under-feeding!

BEHAVIOUR

The general behaviour and temperament of a healthy dog will vary with the breed. At one end of the scale, the small terriers, such as Westies, Cairns and Jack Russells, are very lively, hyperactive little dogs. They are always on the go. Lethargic behaviour would suggest a problem. At the other end of the scale, larger dogs such as the Bloodhound, St Bernard and Great Dane are happy to sleep for most of the day, provided they are exercised in between naps!

Most of us now allow our dogs to live indoors. This is fine, provided they are trained to fit in with the behaviour patterns and hygiene expected from all who live in the house. Due to confusion over which season of the year it is, because our houses

---

NORMAL PARAMETERS

Temperature	38–39°C (100.4–102.2°F)
Heart/pulse rate	70–120 beats per minute
Respiration, at rest	10–30 breaths per minute
panting	up to 200 breaths per minute
Puberty, both sexes	6–8 months
Pregnancy (Gestation period)	63 days
Length of oestrous cycle	18–21 days
Frequency of oestrus	every 6 months
Food requirements, puppy	60g/kg/day ⎱ moist food
adult	30g/kg/day ⎰
Water requirements	40ml/kg/day
Urine output	20ml/kg/day
Frequency of defaecation	1–6 times daily
Red blood cell count	$5.5–8.5 \times 10^{12}$/1 blood
Haemoglobin	12–18g/dl blood
White blood cell count	$6–18 \times 10^{9}$/1 blood

---

2 You and Your Vet

THE VETERINARY SURGEON

All veterinary surgeons have studied at university for at least five years for a veterinary degree before graduating and being accepted as members of the Royal College of Veterinary Surgeons. They are then entitled to place these qualifications after their name. For example BVSc. (Bachelor of Veterinary Science) is one author's qualification from Liverpool University, while the other's is MA, Vet MB, (Master of Art, Bachelor of Veterinary Medicine) from Cambridge University. All the Veterinary Universities award their own degree but there is no difference between them – all recipients are equally qualified. Once a degree is awarded, Membership of the Royal College of Veterinary Surgeons follows and the letters MRCVS are added to the title on payment of an annual retention fee to the Royal College. Only then is the vet able to begin his professional life. In the USA, the degree awarded in all but one university is the DVM (Doctor of Veterinary Medicine).

The university veterinary training course covers all animals from horses, farm animals and poultry, to pet dogs, cats and smaller, children's pets. There is a tremendous amount to learn and to remember, so many vets in practice now tend to treat only certain species, or groups of species, such as horses, farm animals or small animals (pets). There are many alternatives to working in general practice for a veterinary surgeon. Once qualified he, or she, may decide to enter the teaching side of the profession, or research, or work for the Ministry of Agriculture, a pharmaceutical company or one of the animal charities. Another interesting fact is that, nowadays, half of the vets qualifying each year are female. This compares with about one in six some twenty years ago.

Many vets in general practice now are beginning to study for extra qualifications in subjects that are of particular interest to them. This may be in Dermatology (skin diseases), Ophthalmology (eye diseases) or Radiology (X-rays and their interpretation) to name but a few. A very useful referral

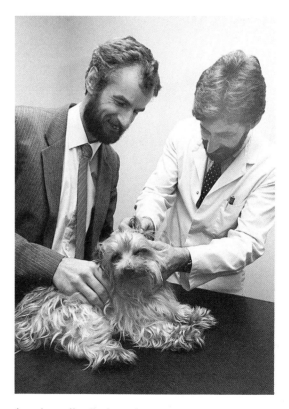

A vet in small-animal practice.

service for particular problem cases for the general practitioner is thus being created.

THE VETERINARY PRACTICE

The titles of veterinary practices may be confusing. Some are named after the veterinary surgeons that own them, while others are called Veterinary Surgery, Veterinary Clinic, Veterinary Centre or even Pet Health Centre. These, in fact, are all the same type of general practice although, of course, the services and facilities offered may vary. In the USA, titles of veterinary practices can also vary. Satellite Clinics provide facilities for outpatients, while hospitals range from Animal Hospitals, Central Hospitals and Animal Medical

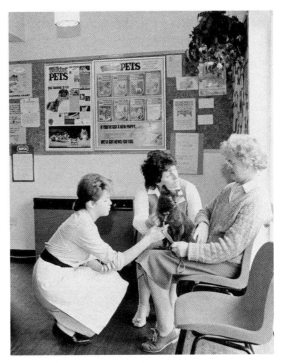

In the waiting room.

Centers to Speciality Hospitals and Emergency Hospitals.

A typical small animal veterinary practice will consist of veterinary surgeons, veterinary nurses and ancillary staff. Some practices, such as our own, will be fairly large (we have seven veterinary surgeons and eleven veterinary nurses in the practice) while others may consist of just one veterinary surgeon and one veterinary nurse. All veterinary practices are required to provide a 24-hour emergency service every day of the year. A large part of your vet's normal working day, however, will be spent dealing with your pet's more routine problems or giving advice on preventive medicine, such as vaccination and worming. In his practice he will have an operating theatre, X-ray facilities, an examination room and dispensary where medicines are stored. In addition, he may have a ward where patients are hospitalised overnight,

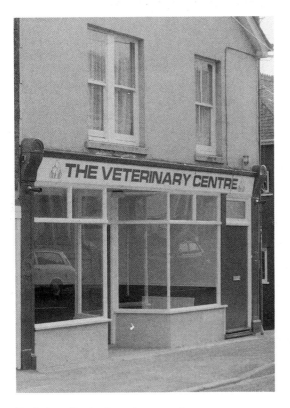

Typical small-animal veterinary practice.

an on-site laboratory to help with diagnosis, and residential facilities for vets or nurses who are on-call.

On arrival at the practice, you should find neat and polite nursing staff, or a receptionist, who will probably be wearing a uniform. Your pet's case history record card should be readily to hand, so that the vet can refer back to previous illnesses and treatments.

Most practices have set surgery times, usually in the morning and evening, and some also have afternoon surgeries. More practices nowadays are offering an appointment system as an alternative to the 'sit and wait your turn' system. Some practices are open for consultations all day by appointment, whilst others even have surgeries on Sundays.

Veterinary Hospitals

You may notice that some veterinary practices are called veterinary hospitals. These, as well as functioning just as all the other types of veterinary practices in the treatment of sick and injured animals, are inspected by the Royal College of Veterinary Surgeons every two years and have a range of facilities and standard of design and construction sufficient to be granted the title veterinary hospital. These facilities include resident nurses or veterinary surgeons on the premises all the time, heated dog and cat wards for long- or short-term patients with arrangements for their sanitary requirements, on-site X-ray facilities, laboratory facilities, fully equipped operating theatres and treatment rooms with shadowless lighting, anaesthetic apparatus and resuscitation equipment. In addition, the construction, design, and wall and floor finishes have to be to a certain standard to minimise spread of disease. Adequate parking facilities also have to be available.

FEES AND SERVICES

The type of veterinary practice you choose will depend on your requirements. Service, personal attention and facilities vary and, of course, so do fees. There are no standard

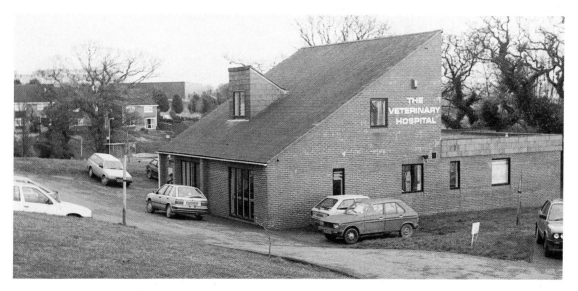

A Veterinary Hospital.

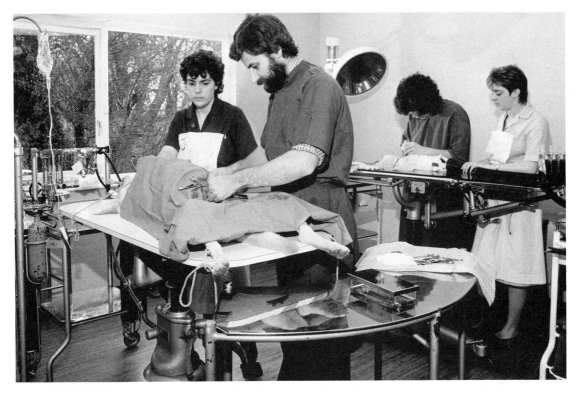

The operating theatre.

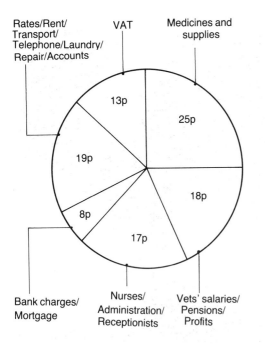

*Fig 2 Breakdown of veterinary costs. Average outgoings
for every £1 of fees received*

veterinary fees. They usually reflect the overheads and level of services being offered, although the geographical location of the practice can also affect them. For example, a city practice is likely to have to charge more than a country one. A practice which has purchased the latest available equipment, such as modern X-ray, diathermy and cryosurgery equipment or ultrasonic dental machines, and has hospitalisation facilities with on-site staff, and an on-site laboratory for rapid diagnosis, will be likely to have higher fees than one offering just the basic services. Your veterinary surgeon has had to purchase and finance his own practice (there are no grants available), so higher fees usually reflect a larger expenditure on equipment or staff to serve you and your pet. Veterinary hospitals tend to be the most expensive but they are regularly inspected to ensure they provide a full and specified range of facilities.

PET HEALTH INSURANCE

The fees charged may affect your choice of practice. However, in making that choice it is important to realise that veterinary medicine is improving all the time and paralleling human medicine. The extra benefits of modern treatment to your dog will cost more and more. There is now, however, no need to worry about fees at all, as there are several reputable pet health insurance companies who will insure your dog against veterinary costs for an annual premium roughly equivalent to a good meal out for two! Third party insurance is also included in case your dog, for instance, damages other people or their property. Taking out pet health insurance is such an obvious thing to do that we cannot understand why at present only about ten per cent of pets are insured. It means that whenever a diagnostic test, treatment, medicine, operation or hospitalisation is

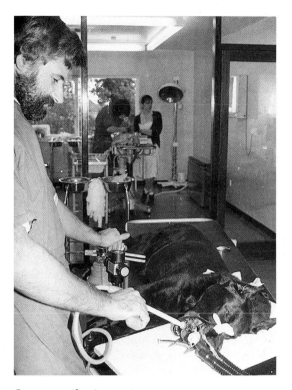

Cryosurgery (freezing) equipment in use on a mouth tumour.

It is usual now for each visit to the surgery to be paid for at the time of attendance. This improves the cash flow of the practice, which helps to keep the fees down as less staff time is spent on accounts. Furthermore, this also allows for greater reinvestment in the practice to the benefit of the patients and their owners alike.

When choosing a veterinary practice, it is important to decide first which type of practice you wish to register with, then ask around the local dog owners for their recommendations. When clients move away from Plymouth, we always suggest they choose their next vet by this method, unless we know a colleague to whom we can refer them.

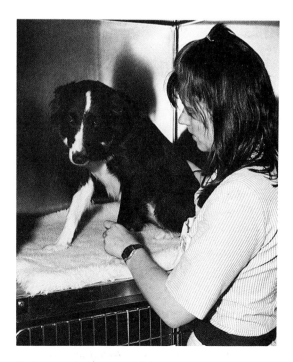

Trainee veterinary nurse with in-patient.

27

needed, your vet can undertake these without the owner having to worry about where the fees are coming from. In other words, it means the patient has the maximum chance of survival. Your veterinary practice will provide full information on the insurance policies available.

REGISTERING WITH A PRACTICE

When you have decided which practice to attend, you should telephone to enquire whether an appointment is necessary, or whether the system is one of open surgeries. You could also enquire whether the practice is willing to carry out house calls, if these are ever needed. It is as well to register your pets with the practice before things go wrong, so that in an emergency you are familiar with the system. A full case history will be kept and updated each time your dog attends. This is of great value in cases of drug allergies, or previous or current treatments, particularly if, for some reason, your usual vet is not available and one of his colleagues attends the case. Loyalty of clients to the practice is very important to vets and equally important for the dog as the case history notes and medical records kept over the years can be extremely important and even lifesaving to the patient.

It is better for all concerned, if you see the same veterinary surgeon each time you attend the surgery. To this end, you should find out when he, or she, normally holds consultations, or enquire before you attend. Gradually, over the years, you develop a relationship (and often the pet does too!) and you should find it easy to communicate your worries and triumphs to your vet. For us, it is not just a job but a vocation, and we like to get to know patients and owners, and follow cases through personally.

Your own vet will also probably prefer to operate on your dog himself, should it ever be necessary. We really do get highly involved with our cases. One of the most rewarding aspects of our way of life is that we can diagnose the illness, administer the medical treatment, take the X-rays and operate if necessary – all within our own surgeries without having to refer the case on to a consultant.

SECOND OPINIONS

There may be occasions when, for various reasons, a second opinion is necessary. Your vet can arrange this for you with a neighbouring practice or a university referral service. You may, on the other hand, just decide you are dissatisfied with the treatment or results. In such a case, you are completely free to seek another vet's advice and opinion but the second vet is bound, by our profession's ethical code, to consult the first vet, prior to seeing the case. This is to safeguard the patient and to ensure that no treatment is given that will cause an adverse reaction to the drugs already in use on the patient. In practice, a second opinion can be of benefit in a difficult case. Both vets should then discuss the case and decide on further action. It is usual for you to be referred back to the original vet for the continuation of the case.

It is, of course, possible for you to change practices either for geographical reasons or through dissatisfaction. At your request, your dog's medical records should be transferred to the new practice. If your dog is actively under treatment, the routine as outlined for second opinions applies.

THE HEALTH EXAMINATION

The clinical examination of your dog differs from that of a human in that the vet cannot ask the dog how it feels or where it hurts! This is often an advantage, as it means we are not given any false or imagined information! So, the first part of the examination consists of history-taking where the vet asks the owner questions about symptoms and behaviour. It is a good idea to write out a list of the things that are worrying you about your dog and take it with you to the surgery. This ensures you will not forget anything when explaining your worries to the vet, and it is of great help to him. An examination of the dog then follows, usually on the consulting room table. The owner may hold the dog gently for this or perhaps a veterinary nurse is called in to help. The exact nature, or extent, of the clinical examination will be determined by the symptoms described by the owner. For example, a dog presented with a vague history of listlessness and lack of appetite will require a full examination including temperature, pulse, chest, examination of eyes, mouth and throat, and palpation of his abdomen. On the other hand, a dog who has suddenly started to scratch his ear may well require merely an examination of this organ to reveal the cause.

This consultation may take from five to twenty minutes, but usually an average of ten minutes is needed to establish a tentative diagnosis, explain the situation and supply treatment for a straightforward case. Sometimes, especially with behavioural problems such as destructive or aggressive dogs, the consultation will take much longer and may even be held at the client's home. At the end of the consultation, the vet will tell you what he thinks the outcome of the case will be (this is called the prognosis). He may refer you and your dog back for a second examination either the next day (if he is particularly worried) or after a few days, or weeks, of treatment. If he recommends that you bring the patient back to the surgery for him to re-examine after a course of treatment, you should ensure that you attend. The vet is the best person to judge whether the illness has cleared up or if further treatment is necessary.

At the end of an examination, many veterinary surgeons will start the treatment by giving an injection. This is for several good reasons. An ill dog will often refuse food, or he may have sickness and diarrhoea, so medicines, which are often given hidden in food, would not be fully utilised. In addition, the injected medicine works more quickly as the drug is absorbed rapidly into the blood stream. This will often mean that by the time the second day's drugs are needed, they will readily be accepted in food or absorbed from the gut. It is fair to say that most dogs are oblivious to the injection – they are not expecting it to hurt and with the modern, disposable syringe and very sharp needle it does not! It is often easier to give an injection than tablets.

With the help of the history and symptoms given by the owner and the findings at the examination of the patient, your vet will often be able to reach a diagnosis or suggest a line of treatment. However, if the cause of the problem is unclear further tests may be necessary. Some conditions, such as diabetes or hip dysplasia, can be diagnosed only after further tests.

DIAGNOSTIC TESTS

Blood tests are useful in the diagnosis of certain conditions, for example, liver or kidney disease, diabetes, certain tumours, anaemias and leukaemia, and various infections. *Urine tests* help in the diagnosis of

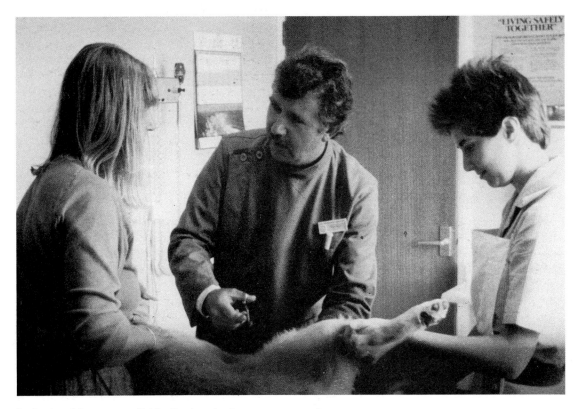

In the consulting room – a Golden Retriever has her sutures removed.

bladder and kidney disease, diabetes and liver problems. *Faeces samples* can identify parasitic worms, bowel disease and pancreatic disease. Sometimes *small skin and hair samples* may be painlessly taken to aid the investigation of skin disorders. *Samples of pus* taken on sterile swabs can be used to identify infections and the antibiotics needed to cure them. All of these tests can be carried out by the surgery staff but some practices prefer to send samples to outside laboratories.

Your dog may need to stay in the surgery for a short while to have some of these tests performed, often under a mild tranquilliser. He will certainly have to stay for a while to have an X-ray taken, if this is deemed necessary for a diagnosis. Many X-rays now have to be taken under a general anaesthetic to comply with the 'Exposure to Radiation' regulations. Some patients have to be admitted into the veterinary hospital, or surgery, just for observation before a definitive diagnosis can be made. However, this is usually far more traumatic for the owner than for the dog! Surprisingly, most dogs settle down well when left at the surgery because they respond well to competent, careful handling.

ANAESTHESIA

Local Anaesthesia

In human medicine, many procedures are carried out under local anaesthesia because once the area to be operated on has lost its sensation, we are content to sit still and behave ourselves! Not so with the dog who

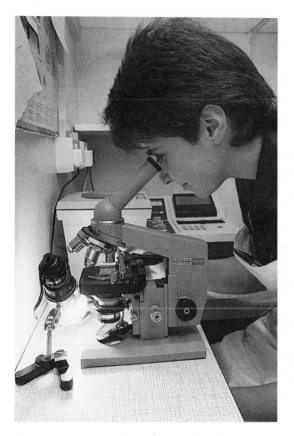

A veterinary nurse examines a skin sample under a microscope.

will struggle and misbehave because it cannot be explained to him that the procedure will not hurt. Thus very few surgical procedures are carried out after an injection of a local anaesthetic alone in small animal practice.

General Anaesthesia

Using modern anaesthetics and modern techniques, general anaesthesia is as safe and successful for dogs as it is for humans. Thus, the vet will often resort to general anaesthesia for the most minor of procedures to ensure the dog does not feel pain or distress or does not panic in unfamiliar surroundings with unfamiliar people.

The procedure is simple and not at all unpleasant for the dog. Ideally he will have been starved for twelve hours to ensure that his stomach is empty of food. However, water must not be withheld. He is then checked over to ensure that he is fit for the anaesthetic, weighed and usually given a premedication injection to sedate him slightly and to dry up his saliva ensuring his airway is clear.

When the time comes for his anaesthetic, he is held gently in the sitting position by a nurse who holds a foreleg up while the vet clips a small area of hair away below the elbow to expose the area of skin where the cephalic vein runs. The vet then injects a measured dose of anaesthetic into the vein and by the count of five, the dog is anaesthetised and lying peacefully on his side. At this stage, an endotracheal tube is inserted gently down his throat to ensure his airway is clear and this is connected to an anaesthetic machine. A minor procedure, such as a tooth extraction or broken nail removal, can be carried out without further anaesthetic, but if the surgical procedure is more major, a gaseous anaesthetic, usually one called fluothane, is administered in combination with oxygen and, on some occasions, nitrous oxide. He can be kept safely under anaesthesia by this method for very long operations during which his condition is constantly monitored by the vet and the nurse.

Recovery is usually smooth and, towards the end of the operation, the anaesthetic is withdrawn and oxygen continued on its own. His previous sedation usually ensures he is not too aware of his surroundings until he is home again.

After routine procedures, most vets aim to discharge the patient the same day, but never until the dog is fully conscious and it is safe for him to go home. If the operation is more serious or complicated, it may be necessary to hospitalise the patient for a day or two until he is fit to return home.

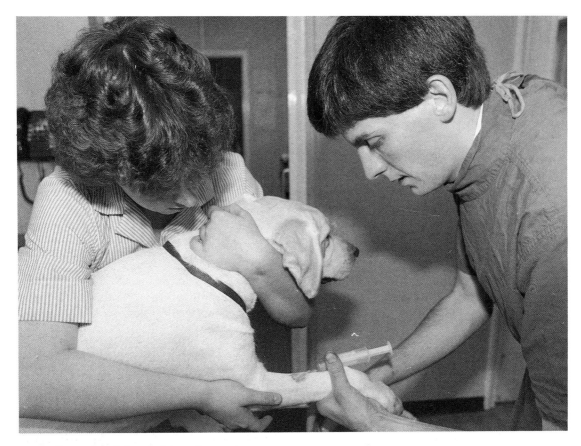

A general anaesthetic being administered to a patient.

RADIOGRAPHY

Radiography is the making of film records, commonly called X-rays, of the internal structures of the body and it is used more for diagnosis of disorders of the locomotor system than any other body system. A diagnostic X-ray picture is obtained when X-rays are projected from an X-ray machine through part of the body on to an X-ray film, which is then developed rather like a photographic film. Where the X-rays are not obstructed, they turn the film black and where a high degree of obstruction occurs, the film remains white. Different tissues of the body absorb differing amounts of X-rays. Bones, for example, absorb far more X-rays than the surrounding muscles so the bone can easily be seen as a white image on the darker surrounds of the X-ray film.

Radiography in veterinary practice is required by law to fulfil all the safety standards that are demanded for human radiography. For example, the vet or nurse must wear protective clothing with a monitor badge, and the X-ray equipment must be in a safe room from which X-rays cannot escape. Very few animals will lie still on an X-ray table, so it is common practice to take X-ray pictures under a short-acting anaesthetic or heavy sedation. This has several advantages. Firstly, it is easier to position the dog because often he is in pain or frightened. Secondly, because the dog is relaxed it is easier to examine the part to be X-rayed. Lastly, the safety of the human operator is paramount and, in most

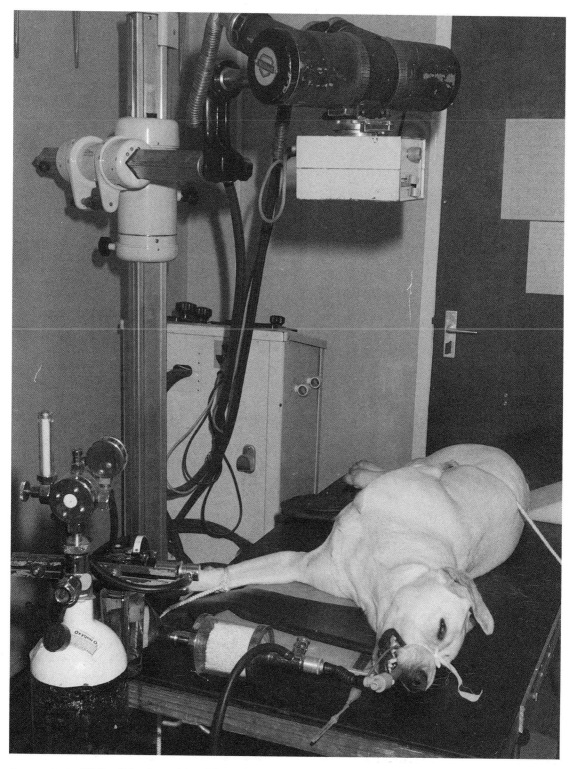

An anaesthetised Yellow Labrador positioned for a left-shoulder X-ray.

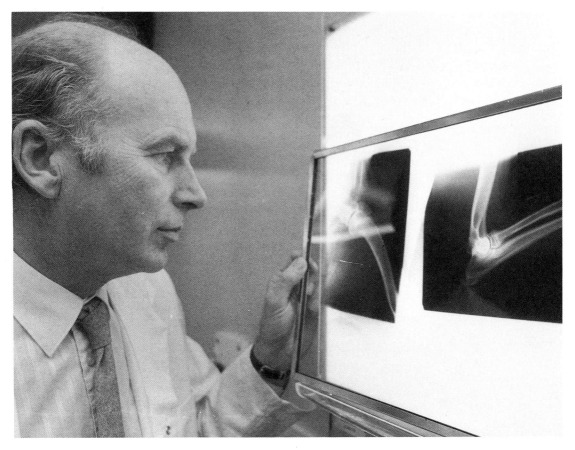

X-rays of a shoulder and elbow under close scrutiny by a vet.

cases, he must be able to leave the room while the X-ray is taken. The law is quite specific as to the circumstances under which X-rays may be taken using manual restraint. Therefore, if your vet advises you that anaesthetic consent is necessary, you must be prepared to give it.

WHEN HELP IS NEEDED

Your veterinary practice is not just a place to contact when you have problems. If you are unsure whether you need to attend, it would be worthwhile making a telephone call to the nurse or receptionist. The vet cannot spend his day answering routine enquiries or he would have no time to treat his patients, but his staff are knowledgeable and trained to help with most enquiries. They will call him to the telephone if it is felt advisable or if they are unsure of the answer to your query.

Your local practice is there to help you – both with problems and with routine enquiries. Where better to telephone or attend for advice on choice of pet, where to get one from or what to look for in a new puppy? Advice is also frequently sought and given on boarding kennels, pet health insurance, feeding, training, behavioural problems, routine worming and flea control.

A day in the life of a small animal veterinary surgeon is full of interest. There will be many routine vaccinations against the killer diseases, and treatment of dogs that have these killer diseases because they were not vaccinated. There will be both routine claw clippings and operations on dogs which have swallowed stones and other foreign bodies. One puppy recently swallowed £20 in notes which, luckily, was more than it cost to retrieve them! There will be complicated road accident cases involving X-rays, transfusions and fracture repair and there will be Caesarean births. All in all, nothing is too simple or complicated for your local veterinary surgeon to help with, so you should not hesitate to telephone or visit if help is needed.

3 The New Puppy

CHOOSING A SUITABLE PUPPY

The National Canine Defence League (NCDL) has coined a slogan which reads 'A dog is for life not just for Christmas'. If you bear this phrase in mind, choosing the right puppy should not be so difficult. Barring accidents or unforeseen problems, your new puppy should live for nine to thirteen years depending on the breed you choose. Therefore, it is necessary to project forward to ensure that you can, and will, care for this new member of the family for that length of time. You may be lucky and have your companion for longer and indeed, we have known just a few dogs live to be twenty years old.

Once you are convinced that you can, and wish to, look after a dog properly for that length of time, the next move is to choose the right breed or type of dog. There are many pure breeds of dog (pedigree) and each breed will grow to a standard size, have a standard type of coat and, within reason, a standard type of behaviour pattern. Thus, it is easier to choose a suitable pet dog from the pedigree breeds if you have certain criteria to fill. This does not mean to say that a mixed breed of dog (mongrel) will not make a good pet. He may well turn out to be the ideal dog for you but you will be unable to predict accurately his size, coat length or behaviour. This may not be important in certain homes, but some idea of these

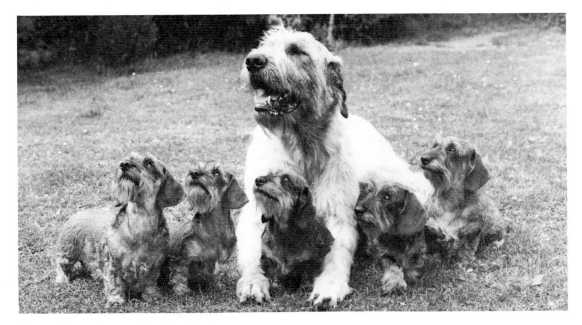

Choose a dog to suit your needs.

variables can be obtained by seeing the dam (mother) and, if possible, or even known, the sire (father) of the puppy. A pedigree form is not a guarantee of health but a guarantee of breed standard.

Your local veterinary surgeon will be able to advise you on the correct choice of dog for your situation. Obviously a large, active, outdoor breed such as a Labrador or a Retriever should not be kept in a small town flat with no garden. They need frequent exercise and plenty of space. If active dogs are confined in too small areas, without enough space to move around in during the day, they become bored and destroy their surroundings, such as furniture and wallpaper. It may not be sufficient to walk them twice a day to prevent this happening. However, some large breeds are not so active and, provided they are exercised regularly in open spaces, they may be relatively happy in a small house. Other problems, however, then arise. Large dogs eat large meals and produce large stools. These should not be deposited on public highways, pathways or parks unless they are disposed of immediately by the owner with a 'poop-scoop' device, or similar. This can be a real problem in a flat or house with no garden or yard. All dogs should be trained to relieve themselves in the owner's garden or yard and only be taken out for exercise.

Generally, small breeds suit small homes. A Yorkshire Terrier, King Charles Spaniel, Toy Poodle or Miniature Dachshund, for example, would make an ideal pet for a person or family in a small or normal sized home where the dog may have reasonable exercise, but not too much space. A Labrador, Springer or Cocker Spaniel, Setter or Boxer, for instance, would be a good choice for a person or family with a reasonable sized home and garden, who also enjoy taking long, daily walks with their dog. These breeds are suitable for the active person who loves walking on the moors,

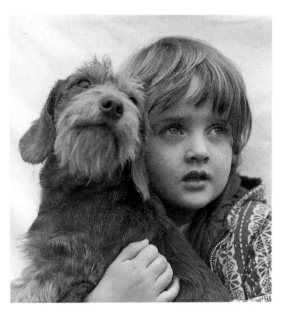

A Miniature Wire-Haired Dachshund makes an ideal family pet.

beaches or in the countryside. If you own a large house and garden, where the dog can wander safely and freely, perhaps a giant breed such as an Irish Wolfhound, Great Dane or Rottweiler may suit you. However, you should remember the extra cost of feeding this size of dog.

It is also necessary to consider the amount of time you have available for grooming. A short-coat breed, such as a Boxer, will merely need a quick brush most days, whereas an Old English Sheepdog or Afghan Hound will need considerably more time spent on grooming. An hour a day is a reasonable estimate – more if he has just exercised in the rain through the local woods! Many dogs of these breeds end up at the vet's to be dematted under a sedative or general anaesthetic.

Food is an important consideration. A toy breed will cost very little to feed each day while an active large breed, eating 1–1½kg (2–3lb) of meat daily may cost five to ten times more, depending on your choice of food. Thus, food costs for a large

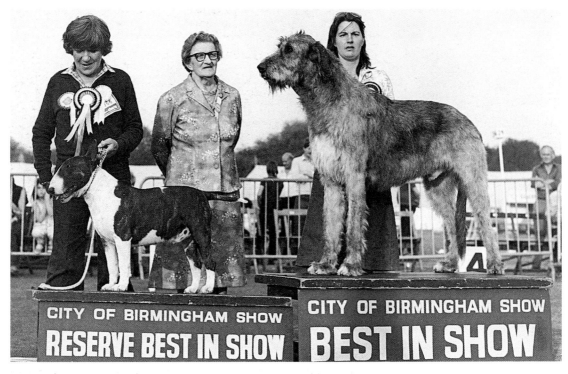

Proud owner – breeders at a Dog Show.

breed must be taken into consideration before acquiring a dog of this type.

As your new dog will be a member of your family for some considerable time, it is essential to look at your life style and home from the dog's point of view. An active little terrier, or gundog breed, will be in his element living with an active, boisterous family, but a quiet toy breed, such as a Poodle or Pomeranian, could have a very unhappy life in such a situation. A Bloodhound will be none too happy to be woken up frequently by hyperactive young children, whereas a Boxer will be upset if left alone too long!

The most important ingredient for success is time. You must have time available to spend with your dog, and initially, when he is a puppy, he will take up much more of your time. Unless you will be with him frequently, there is no point starting a relationship at all.

SOURCES OF PEDIGREE AND MONGREL DOGS

Dog Breeding Kennels

These kennels usually specialise in one or two breeds and a recommendation from your local vet, or other satisfied customers, is essential.

Individual Owner-Breeders

One or two dogs are owned and bred as a hobby by an individual owner–breeder. This is a good source, as puppies raised in this fashion are used to family life when you buy them. However, a recommendation from someone you trust is advisable.

Stray-Dog Homes

These homes will supply not only puppies, but also adult dogs, which, for one reason

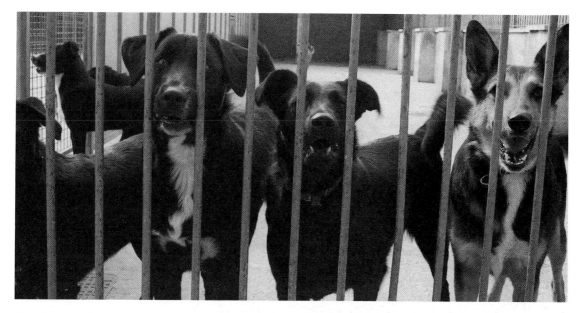

Dogs in a stray-dog home.

or another, had a previous unsatisfactory home. These dogs need good homes and usually have been cared for well while on the premises. Disease or predetermined behaviour patterns may be a potential problem. This is usually the cheapest source of dogs and, surprisingly, pedigree dogs are often available.

Puppy Farms

These are literally large-scale dog breeding farms. Puppies are not usually sold direct to the public but to dealers, who then sell them on at a profit.

Dog Dealers

Dog dealers usually trade as a large kennels supplying many different breeds of dog, few of which are born on the premises. They buy in puppies from owners who cannot, or do not, sell them or from puppy farms. Then the dealers sell the puppies on to the public. Recommendation is essential, but it can be a useful visit to see different breeds. However, a visit to a dealer does

encourage impulse buying, so it is preferable to visit one or more local dog shows to see the various breeds in more normal circumstances.

There are some basic rules to be followed if you wish to stand a maximum chance of purchasing the ideal dog for you.

1 Never be in a hurry or impatient to make the purchase.
2 Ensure that the puppy is from a reliable source, is fit and well, and will suit you. It is far better to wait for the right dog than to rush in and buy the first one of your chosen breed that becomes available.
3 If possible, purchase a puppy from the premises where he was born. There are several advantages in doing this. You will be able to examine and assess the size and temperament of the dam (and possibly also the sire). The puppy will not have been subjected to the stress of a journey from his original home and he will not have had his behaviour modified by anyone prior to you. You should, therefore, be able to gain an impression from the breeder and his

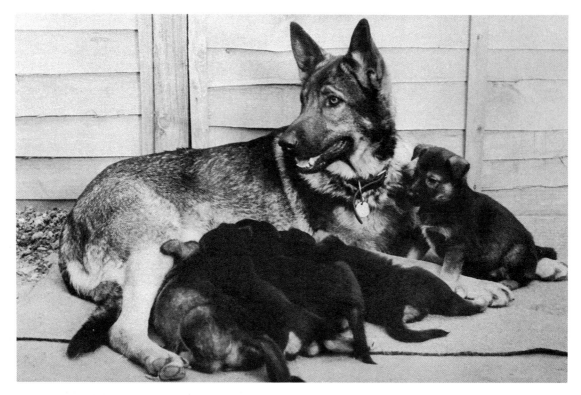

A healthy litter of German Shepherd puppies.

premises as to the quality of the puppy. In addition, the puppy is less likely to be incubating any disease.

AGE OF PURCHASE

Do not buy the puppy until he is at least six weeks old. The ideal age is from six to ten weeks, depending on his size, his health and your circumstances. There is evidence to show that this is the best age for puppies to adapt to their new life style and owners.

If your choice is to be a pedigree puppy, check with your veterinary surgeon whether there are any inherited disease problems that you should avoid with that breed. This may mean, for instance, ensuring that the dam and sire are free from hip dysplasia or inherited eye disease. This simple step can save you years of disappointment and

heartache with a lame, crippled or blind dog. If the breeder cannot give you this assurance, then buy your puppy elsewhere.

Also, why not ask your vet to recommend sources of particular breeds? He is likely to know the better local breeders or a caring one-dog owner whose bitch has just had a litter.

There are both advantages and disadvantages in purchasing an adult dog from one of the many stray homes and rescue centres which offer dogs for re-homing. On the positive side, you will know the size, coat type, and, to some degree, the temperament of the dog. The staff at the home should be able to tell you whether the dog will fit in with your way of life; they are caring people who wish the dog well in the future. However, it is possible that the adult dog may not be toilet trained as no one has been available to teach him and he may rapidly ruin your home. He may be used to a busy household around him and the peace of your home may bore him. Bored dogs can become destructive. He may not be trained to a lead or come when called. However, most stray homes will allow you to have a dog on a trial basis for a while, for you to assess his suitability. One thing is certain – the dog is in great need of a caring home.

In general, you should never purchase a dog on impulse and, wherever possible, seek a recommendation from others. Do not accept a dog with a known behavioural problem thinking that he will be different in your home – he is unlikely to change.

WHAT TO LOOK FOR IN THE NEW PUPPY

Once you have decided on the breed of dog you require, and the source, you are ready to choose your own puppy. What do you look for? Look at the dam first. She will give you an indication of how your puppy will be when adult, both in looks and temperament. Take a look at her away from her puppies; she may be protective when they are around.

Choose a puppy that is interested in you. It may not necessarily be the young leader that gets to you first – that one may be too dominant for you – but it should certainly not be the one that cowers in the corner. Never choose one that you feel sorry for. Life with your dog will be miserable if the puppy grows into a dog that refuses to socialise with people or other dogs.

Check that he is in good bodily condition. Make sure he is bright and alert, not too thin and that he has no discharge from his eyes or nose. His ears should be responsive to sounds. The coat should be glossy, and there should be no sores, bald patches or scabs on his skin. Observe the puppy in his pen, both to assess activity and the way he moves. Make sure there is no obvious

lameness and check all his legs are sound and straight. Look around the pen to ensure there are no signs of diarrhoea or vomit and that none of the puppies looks unwell or is showing obvious signs of illness, such as coughing.

MANAGEMENT AND CARE OF THE NEW ARRIVAL

Bedding

Before the puppy is brought into his new home, there are some purchases and arrangements that have to be made. A bed should be waiting for him. Puppies chew a lot and so a cardboard box with a blanket is better than a wicker or plastic bed at this age. New synthetic bedding materials which can be washed and dried are available. You can then progress to a more conventional bed, basket or beanbag as he gets older.

Feeding

A food bowl and a water bowl should be waiting for your new puppy. Check with the breeder which type of food the puppy is used to and make sure you have some ready for his arrival at his new home. The breeder should supply each new owner with a diet sheet so make certain you ask for one. His water bowl should always be full of clean water.

Collar and Lead

If you tell the pet shop what breed of dog you are buying, they will advise you on the correct collar and lead. He will probably need several collars of varying sizes as he grows up. Remember to buy his identity disc which is obtainable at pets shops or most key cutting kiosks. Discs are better than screw-top name containers which often unscrew and fall off.

Toys

It is a good idea to purchase safe, non-toxic toys that your puppy can chew without swallowing. A large, raw, marrow bone from a butcher is ideal as are chew sticks or other tough, safe, indestructible chewy toys. If these are provided for your puppy to chew on, your furniture and carpets will be less liable to damage!

Vaccinations

Check with the breeder whether the puppy has received any vaccinations and if so, when. If he has, the breeder should provide you with a vaccination certificate and advise you when the next injection is due.

Worming

Ask the breeder when the puppy was last wormed. Your vet is certain to ask you as this should be carried out at fortnightly intervals up to the age of three months.

Pedigree Certificate

If you have purchased a pedigree puppy, you should be supplied with his certificate when you collect him. This shows his ancestry.

Pet Health Insurance

Ask if the breeder has taken out a temporary health insurance policy to cover any un-expected problems in the first six weeks. The better breeders do this for you and we advise you to continue with it. If the puppy is not insured, ask your vet for details at the first health examination and vaccination.

The Homecoming

For the journey back home with your new puppy, remember to take a blanket to keep him warm, a kitchen roll in case he is travel sick, and, if you are travelling alone to fetch him, transport him in an escape-proof basket. It is preferable for someone to accompany you so that one of you is free to comfort and cuddle him in the car on his new adventure.

Remember that the first night with you will be his first ever night alone. It is, therefore, a good idea to collect him in the morning, if you can, so he has a longer time to adapt to his new surroundings and to get to know you before it is bedtime.

THE FIRST FEW DAYS

A new puppy will instantly alter your life! There will be upsets and delights as he messes and chews, learns a new trick or enjoys playing with you. It is important to realise that his life has been totally altered too, from one of complete security with his mother, litter mates, and familiar humans, to a life where he is suddenly on his own with a strange family in unfamiliar surroundings. This can be very stressful and, initially, he will probably whine at night. Usually, however, this is transient and ceases once the puppy realises he is, in fact, secure and that his new friends are always there when he wakes up. It may be necessary to bring his bed into your bedroom for a few nights but it is better to battle it out and leave him on his own. Leaving a dim light on in his room overnight may help. It can be counter-productive to get up and comfort him as this reward may encourage him to cry. It is much better to ignore him, or voice a slight reprimand each time.

In our experience, puppies may have a little diarrhoea during the first few days in their new home. This will clear up by withholding food and milk for twenty-four hours and then feeding a light diet of chicken, fish or scrambled egg until the problem is resolved. The possibility of diarrhoea can be minimised by feeding the puppy the same diet that the breeder was using. If the problem persists, or if any untoward signs develop, you should contact your veterinary surgeon for advice.

It is much more likely that your new puppy will be healthy, with bouts of ceaseless energy interspersed with sudden periods of deep sleep. This is completely normal but it may take you by surprise. It is equally likely that he will get the timing wrong. He may collapse in a deep sleep just as you want to play with him and then be at his most active at 11 p.m. when you are ready to go to bed. Patience is essential – his biological clock will correct itself in time!

FEEDING YOUR NEW PUPPY

It is necessary to feed a balanced diet during your puppy's growing period and also during his adult life. This means he will be fed the correct amount of protein, carbohydrate, fat, minerals and vitamins. All these will be provided in the normal course of events if a balanced mixture of foods is given. It should be realised from the outset that although meat is thought of as the natural food of the dog, it only provides some of the daily requirements. If it is fed to the exclusion of other items serious harm can result. Meat is low in carbohydrate but, most important of all, it is very low in minerals and vitamins.

For the first few weeks after purchase, from about eight to fourteen weeks of age, the puppy should continue to have milk, or milk substitute, twice a day in addition to his solid foods. Milk remains the ideal food for the growing animal, for it is rich in easily assimilated protein, fats, carbohydrates and minerals, particularly calcium which is so necessary for bone formation.

As time passes, the puppy will drink less and less milk and eat more and more solid food. At no time should meat alone be given as many puppies, having tasted meat, begin to refuse other foods. As a result, his appetite may deteriorate due to lack of appetite promoting vitamins, particularly the B group, which are almost non-existent in meat.

As soon as solid food is taken, it should consist of half lightly cooked meat, or tinned puppy food, and half cereal foods such as wholemeal bread, prepared puppy meal, cooked vegetables, greens or carrots. A little flavouring, such as Marmite (rich in vitamin B), and a balanced vitamin/ mineral complex may be added to the meal but care should be taken not to exceed the manufacturers' recommended levels. At first, the solid food should be well moistened but this additional fluid should be reduced gradually and withdrawn by the time the puppy is six to seven months old.

It is now possible to obtain complete puppy foods, in dried form, which are fed to the exclusion of everything else except water, of course, which must be available at all times. The choice of diet for your new puppy will depend on many factors, not the least of which is his own preference. Diets should be discussed with your vet at the first puppy consultation.

A young puppy should be fed little and often, like a baby. The number of meals is gradually decreased so that the puppy should have only two meals a day by six to seven months of age.

Weaning to Three Months

Feed four times a day. Two meals should be of milk, or milk and cereal, and two should be semi-solid consisting of meat – either canned puppy food or fresh meat minced or finely cut – lightly cooked and mashed very small. An equal amount of puppy meal or cereal should be added to each meat meal with a copious amount of gravy.

Three to Six Months

At three months leave out one milk meal, and feed one milky meal and two semi-solid meat meals as before. The size of each meal should be increased as the puppy grows. From four months of age, you may continue to feed your puppy three times a day or, by leaving out a meat meal, reduce the meals to two a day. The meat may now be fed in larger pieces with more puppy meal or mixer biscuit with vegetables. A large, raw, beef marrow bone and some hard dog biscuits, which are not small enough to be swallowed whole, may be introduced at this stage to help develop the jaws. Bones of veal, lamb, pork, ham and poultry should be avoided as they crunch easily and may be swallowed in pieces. Cooked bones should never be fed.

It is not wise to feed adult canned dog foods or starchy cereals to puppies under five months of age as this may cause digestive upsets and loss of condition. Good, canned puppy foods and dried complete diets are available.

Over Six Months

Most dogs are fed once daily, usually in the evening, although many continue to take milk, or a small breakfast, in the morning. The puppy biscuit should be changed to mixer biscuit, or terrier or hound meal, depending upon the size of the dog. However, the proportion of meat should not be changed and amounts should be assessed on the basis of weight rather than volume.

As dogs vary in size, from Chihuahuas to Irish Wolfhounds, it is not possible to generalise on the actual amount of food to be given. Puppies should be fed the amount that satisfies them and a good approximate rule is to give 60g (2oz) of food per 1kg (2lb) body weight daily where fresh or canned meat is used as the base.

Adults who require food for maintainance only need approximately 30g (1oz) of food per 1kg (2lb) body weight.

THE FIRST VETERINARY INSPECTION

This will normally be carried out at the time of the first vaccination of the puppy at eight to ten weeks of age. If your new puppy is lively and playful in between naps, eats well and has no obvious signs of illness, it may not be necessary to have a veterinary inspection before the first vaccination is due. If, however, there is anything which causes you concern it would be advisable to take him to your local vet, or at least telephone for advice. It is wise to sort out any problems, which may have been present at the time of purchase, with the breeder as soon as possible.

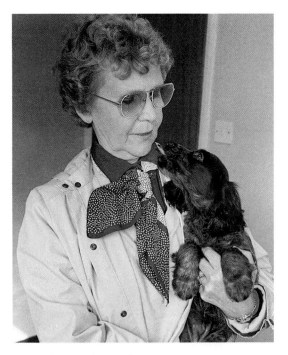

Vaccination time for a Cocker Spaniel puppy.

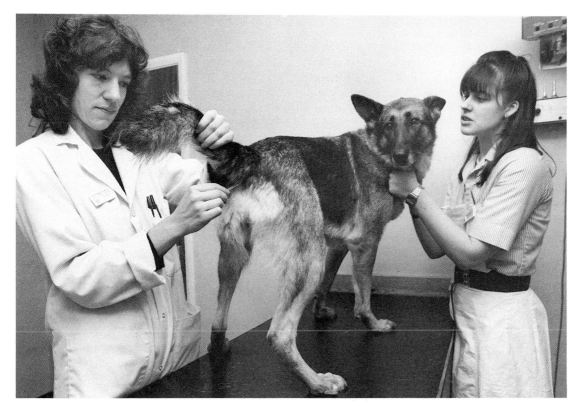

A patient has his temperature taken.

Before vaccinating the puppy, your vet will ensure that he is fit and healthy and able to respond to the vaccination. He will check his temperature, heart and pulse, lungs, eyes, mouth, ears, abdomen and general overall condition. He will, of course, ask you questions about his health and behaviour and will check the puppy for any obvious faults or defects. Unless you have noticed anything unusual it is, of course, highly likely that your puppy will be completely fit and well. However, there are a few problems that may be identified at the first inspection.

The Head

Examination of the head will reveal whether the puppy has a congenital or hereditary problem in this area and there are a few defects that are occasionally seen. Hare lip and cleft palate are problems caused by the centre of the upper roof of the mouth failing to join completely during development in the uterus. Hare lip is seen as a split in the upper lip, extending up to the nostrils. It is unsightly but unlikely to cause the puppy problems, unless he is severely affected. Your veterinary surgeon may later be able to correct this surgically. Cleft palate is an opening in the roof of the mouth which connects with the nose so that food and drink will run back down the nose. This can be a serious problem and difficult to correct.

The upper and lower jaw should be the same length. Any deviation from this is abnormal. If the lower jaw is longer than the upper jaw it protrudes so that the lower incisor teeth jut out in front of the upper teeth. This jaw is said to be undershot. Where the upper jaw is longer than the lower jaw, this is referred to as overshot. Puppies that are affected may well live a normal life but they will not win any major dog shows.

In some breeds of dog the bones on the top of the skull occasionally fail to unite, leaving a small gap called the fontanelle. The brain is, therefore, not fully protected from trauma and the defect is undesirable. In our experience, it occurs most commonly in Chihuahuas but the gap usually closes before maturity.

More commonly, your vet will find minor problems such as mild ear or eye infections that you may not have noticed. He will provide you with any treatment that he considers necessary.

The Chest

An examination of the chest by stethoscope may reveal a heart defect such as valvular disease, or congenital oddities like a hole in the heart or persistent extra arteries where they leave the heart. Fortunately, problems like this are extremely uncommon.

The Abdomen

Palpation (examination by touch) of the abdomen may reveal abnormalities or indicate an infestation of parasitic roundworms. Certainly, any unusual bowel obstructions will be noticed at this stage, as will hernias. In male puppies, the presence of both testicles can often be confirmed at a young age.

Temperature

This may be taken using a well lubricated thermometer inserted gently into the anus. If the temperature is raised, this may be an indication to the vet that the puppy has an infection. A thorough clinical examination should reveal the exact nature of the problem.

In addition to the detailed examination of the various areas described, the vet will assess the general appearance and condition of the puppy. He will note any abnormality of the coat due to deficiencies or parasites, or any abnormalities of the feet, legs and tail. Your vet will be assessing your puppy's condition from the time you enter the room so that the detailed examination may only take a few moments and not distress the puppy, or you, at all. If all is well, he will then progress to the vaccination of the puppy.

VACCINATION OF THE NEW PUPPY

Vaccination is the administration of a modified live, or killed form of an infection which does not cause illness in the puppy. Instead, it stimulates the formation of protecting antibodies against the disease itself. This immunity against a disease is called 'active immunity'. The only other way a puppy can obtain active immunity is by surviving a bout of a disease, but as he cannot be guaranteed survival, vaccination is preferable. This active immunity takes over from the antibodies given to him by his dam in her colostrum, or first milk (called 'passive immunity'), which usually disappear by twelve weeks of age.

There are four major killer diseases against which all puppies should be vaccinated. These are *canine distemper* (also called hardpad), *infectious canine hepatitis*, *leptospirosis* and *canine parvovirus*. In many countries, vaccination against *rabies* is carried out, but not in Great Britain, where this disease has not occurred since 1908. These diseases are described in detail in Chapter 5.

The vaccination course varies according to the type of vaccine used, the age of the puppy and the prevalence of disease in the area in which the puppy lives. Canine

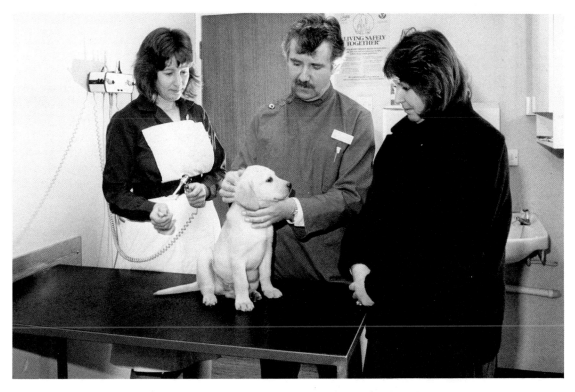

Vaccination time for an eight-week-old Yellow Labrador puppy.

distemper vaccine is a live vaccine and one injection at twelve weeks of age, or over, is sufficient to give immunity for at least one year. Hepatitis vaccine is available in both live and dead forms. As with distemper vaccination, one injection of the live vaccine at twelve weeks or older is all that is needed. Many vets prefer the dead vaccine and using this, two injections, one at eight to ten weeks and the second at twelve weeks, or over, are given. Leptospirosis, again using a dead vaccine, is also given in two injections. One is given at eight to ten weeks, and the second at twelve weeks or over.

Canine parvovirus vaccine is available in both live and dead forms. If the live vaccine is used, the twelve week dose may give adequate immunity until the first booster vaccination at about fifteen months of age. The dead vaccine, preferred by many practices, requires a further dose to be given at sixteen to twenty weeks of age, to ensure satisfactory immunisation. This disease has been so widespread and virulent since its origin in the late 1970s, that puppies usually have an earlier vaccination as well, at six to ten weeks of age.

This may sound complicated but, as the vaccines are combined together, basically the puppy should have two injections two to four weeks apart, starting any time after eight weeks of age. Some ten days or so after the second vaccine, he should have sufficient immunity to be taken out for walks. If the parvovirus vaccine was a dead one, then he should have a further vaccination at sixteen to twenty weeks of age. Thereafter, the current recommendations are that all dogs should have a booster against all four infections each year of their life. This is given in combined form as a single injection.

4 The Growing Dog

This chapter describes disease problems in the puppy between the age of eight weeks, the age at which most owners acquire their new puppy, and maturity, at about one year of age. This is the period in a dog's life when growth is very rapid and certain specific problems occur during this phase, especially in the larger breeds.

DIETARY PROBLEMS

The growing puppy requires a greater intake of food for his size than the adult and it is important that all the nutrients are present in the right amounts (*see* Chapter 3, pages 43–4 for details). Some growing puppies can have enormous appetites but it is important not to let them become overweight as this can affect their bone development. Underfeeding will produce a thin, poorly developed puppy with a ravenous appetite, who may then swallow foreign objects. The best guide to a dog's weight is how he looks and the ease with which his ribs and spine can be felt. In general, a dog that feels very bony is underweight and if the ribs cannot be felt, the dog is overweight.

PROBLEMS OF THE BONES AND JOINTS

Nutritional diseases are now very uncommon as most owners feed one of the many manufactured diets which contain all the necessary nutrients in the right proportions. Deficiency diseases only occur when the owner makes up his own diet incorrectly for the puppy or misunderstands the feeding instructions when using prepared food.

Rickets

This disease, seen very rarely now, is caused by a diet which is low in calcium, phosphorus and vitamin D; it would be a poor cereal diet without milk and meat. Rickets affects the areas of the bone where growth occurs, the growth plates. These become swollen, the bones weak and bowed and the joints distorted. The puppy will be thin and small for his size. On an X-ray the bones appear thin walled and the growth plates thicker than normal.

Treatment The puppy's condition can be improved by feeding the correct diet but the existing distortion of the legs will remain.

Juvenile Osteoporosis

This condition is more common than rickets and is usually caused by an excessive amount of meat in the diet, at the expense of milk and cereal food. Such a diet is rich in phosphorus but poor in calcium. An affected puppy is generally well developed but the bones become thin and weak. There will be varying degrees of lameness and, sometimes, the front legs are bowed. If a bone becomes very weak it may collapse due to a folding fracture. This leads to a deformed, painful limb and a severely lame puppy. Juvenile osteoporosis is diagnosed by an X-ray of the bones and an investigation of the diet.

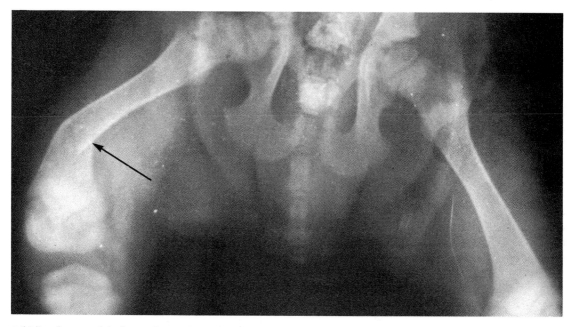

A folding fracture of the femur of a puppy with osteoporosis.

Treatment The condition can be reversed by correcting the diet, but any fractures will need temporary support and the bone will remain deformed.

Hypertrophic Osteodystrophy

This is an uncommon disease of the larger breeds and is seen at about three to six months of age. It was originally thought to be due to vitamin C deficiency but other factors are now considered to be involved, particularly over-supplementation with minerals and vitamins during the growing phase. The affected dog is very miserable, has a high temperature and his joints are very swollen and painful so he is reluctant to move. Distinctive changes can be seen on an X-ray of the bones.

Treatment The disease is usually self-limiting but treatment with large doses of vitamin C may reduce the pain. All vitamin and mineral supplements should be withdrawn and the affected dog fed on a complete balanced diet. If this fails then pain-killing tablets will often be prescribed. The dog can be left with a thickening and deformity of the joints.

Growth Plate Problems

The growth plate (described in greater detail in Chapter 12, page 143) is a thin line of cartilage near the end of each bone. In the young dog bones grow by increasing in length at the growth plate. When the bone ceases to grow, the growth plate disappears. This area is a point of weakness and can easily be damaged. Severe damage to the growth plate may result in shortening or deformity of the bone.

An example of a growth-plate problem is Carpus Valgus in the front legs of (usually) the larger breeds. The leg very noticeably begins to deviate outwards at the carpus or wrist, and immediate surgery is necessary to correct this fault.

Treatment Surgery will be required to straighten the limb. This growth deformity can occur in the hind legs but it is far less

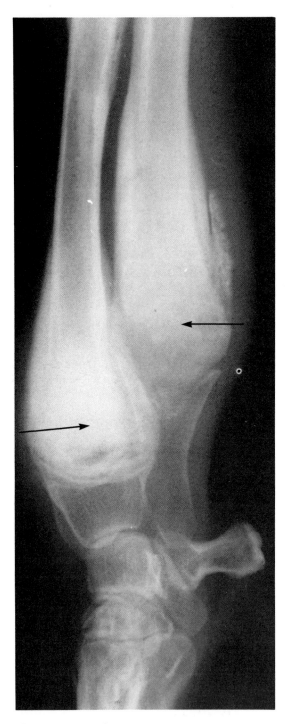

Hypertrophic osteodystrophy in a Great Dane. The radius (left) and ulna (right) are affected at the carpus.

common. In puppies it is not uncommon for bones to fracture at the growth plate. Accurate fixation of the fracture is necessary to prevent abnormal growth of the bone.

There is growing evidence that many of the bone diseases in this age-group are caused by the rapid weight gain encouraged in the larger breeds. The most common mistakes are generally over feeding, especially with protein foods, and over supplementation of the diet with calcium and vitamin D. Protein foods should not exceed twenty-five per cent of the diet and calcium no more than two per cent of the dry matter of the food.

FRONT LEG LAMENESS

The larger breeds seem particularly prone to front leg lameness which may either develop slowly over several weeks, or may suddenly appear after a minor accident. The lameness may be intermittent, the puppy being affected some days but not others, or it may be persistent. During the first examination your vet may check that the diet is correct and then possibly prescribe pain-killing tablets and a period of rest. If, after several weeks, the lameness persists or deteriorates the vet may recommend X-rays to establish if one of the following is present:

Ununited Anconeal Process

This is seen most often in the German Shepherd Dog at around five months of age. It is characterised by pain and a slight enlargement of the elbow joint. An X-ray will show that a small piece of bone in the elbow joint, the anconeal process, has not fused correctly to the ulna. The condition may be present in one or both elbows.

Treatment This small piece of bone must

be removed surgically to relieve the pain and prevent the development of arthritis.

Osteochondritis Dissicans

This disease is more common in the shoulder joints of Rottweilers, Great Danes and Wolfhounds but also occurs in other joints and other breeds. The lameness starts between six and nine months of age and is caused by a piece of cartilage in the joint breaking away from the underlying bone. Usually both shoulders are affected, but one to a greater degree than the other. An X-ray is necessary to demonstrate the defect in the cartilage.

Treatment In severe cases, an operation is performed to remove the loose fragment. If the condition is untreated the joint may become arthritic or the piece of cartilage may become detached and move around in the joint, causing great pain.

Ununited Coronoid Process

The coronoid process is a very small piece of bone at the front of the elbow joint, which causes pain and lameness if it fails to fuse to the ulna. This condition is very difficult to diagnose as the fragment of bone is too small to visualise clearly on an X-ray. However, an ununited coronoid process should be suspected in any young dog whose elbow shows evidence of early arthritis.

Treatment It may be necessary to explore the joint surgically for evidence of an ununited coronoid process and, if present, it should be removed. If untreated the mobile fragment will result in a permanently arthritic joint.

Despite extensive investigation of some cases of front leg lameness in the young dog, no diagnosis as to the cause of the

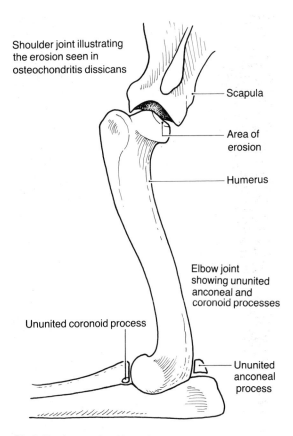

Shoulder joint illustrating the erosion seen in osteochondritis dissicans

Scapula

Area of erosion

Humerus

Elbow joint showing ununited anconeal and coronoid processes

Ununited coronoid process

Ununited anconeal process

Fig 3 Developmental problems of the foreleg

lameness can be made. In our experience, this is especially so in the Labrador. Any non-specific lameness is treated with pain-killing tablets and strict rest, and after several weeks or months the lameness will usually disappear.

HIND LEG LAMENESS

Once again, the larger breeds are more commonly affected due to the extra stresses placed on the growing bones.

Hip Dysplasia

This condition, which is not confined to the growing puppy, is considered in greater detail in Chapter 12 (*see* page 156). The breeds most likely to be affected are the German Shepherd Dog, Old English Sheepdog, Labrador and Retriever. Both the age of onset and the disability caused vary, depending on the degree of deformity of the hip joint.

Symptoms can appear in puppies as young as four or five months of age and are very variable. The puppy may have difficulty standing up from a sitting position, may be reluctant or unable to jump, may walk with a crouch or be unwilling to go for a walk. When he runs, the hind legs may show a peculiar swaying or hopping movement.

A vet presented with a puppy showing the above symptoms will usually carry out further investigations to make a definite diagnosis of hip dysplasia. The puppy will often be examined under an anaesthetic to permit a thorough manipulation of the joint, as the laxity in hip dysplasia can only be felt when the puppy is completely relaxed. At the same time, an X-ray of the hips will be taken.

Treatment In mildly affected dogs it is often sufficient to ensure that the diet is correct, the puppy does not become overweight and that he is given moderate exercise only. This may allow the joints to stabilise. In more severe cases, or where the above treatment has failed, surgery may be required to correct the disability. No puppy suffering from hip dysplasia should be considered as future breeding stock as the condition is known to be hereditary.

Femoral Head Necrosis

This is an uncommon, degenerative disease of the hip joint and it is seen in the smaller breeds, especially the Jack Russell Terrier. The lameness begins at around nine months of age and slowly worsens until the puppy continuously carries the affected leg. Severe

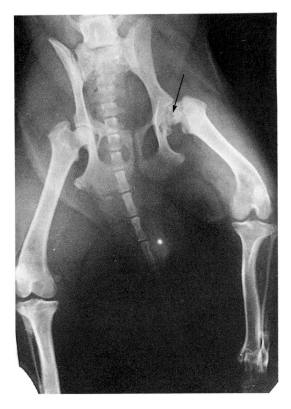

Femoral Head Necrosis of the left hip of a Jack Russell Terrier.

muscle wastage often occurs giving the thigh a very thin appearance. The disease affects the head of the femur causing it to become soft and collapse leaving the hip grossly misshapen. These changes can be seen on an X-ray of the hip.

Treatment Anti-inflammatory drugs, anabolic steroids and/or rest may be all that is required in early mild cases. However, in advanced cases, surgical removal of the diseased part of the bone is the treatment of choice. This is called excision arthroplasty.

Dislocating Patella (Kneecap)

This is a common condition of some of the smaller breeds but is not confined to the young growing dog. An intermittent lameness is produced. When the kneecap slips out of position, the dog carries the leg. After a few paces the kneecap often returns to its normal position and the dog stops limping. This laxity in the ligaments supporting the patella can be felt by the vet on a clinical examination.

Treatment Surgical shortening of the ligaments is usually successful but, in severe cases, the trochlear groove in which the patella runs must be deepened. Very occasionally a projection of bone, the tibial crest, must be repositioned to correct the pull of the ligaments on the patella.

NERVOUS DISEASES

There are an increasing number of inherited diseases affecting the proper functioning of the spinal nerves in young puppies. These diseases are seen in many breeds and include Cairn Terrier storage disease, progressive axonopathy in the Boxer, myelomalacia in the Afghan Hound and swimmers in the Irish Setter. The symptoms appear between three and six months of age and can include a slowly developing weakness of the hind legs, sometimes the front legs, an inability to stand up, incoordination, loss of vision and tremors. There is, unfortunately, no treatment. Most of these diseases are progressive and the dog is usually put to sleep due to developing paralysis.

HEART PROBLEMS

Very few puppies are born with heart defects but when these do occur, they can vary from defective valves to holes in the wall of the heart, which separates the right and left chambers. The age of onset and severity of symptoms will depend on the type of heart problem. In some puppies the defective heart will affect growth from the moment of birth; in other cases heart failure may not occur until eighteen months to two years. On the other hand, the defect may be so insignificant that the affected dog will live a full and normal life. A puppy affected at an early age will be smaller than his litter mates, will be thin and may have a swollen abdomen due to ascites. He will be less inclined to run around and will tire easily. His gums and tongue may be a bluish colour instead of pink, due to lack of oxygen.

When the vet listens to the puppy's heart he may hear a heart murmur. This is a descriptive term for the sound caused by the blood flowing unevenly through the damaged part of the heart. The heart may also sound louder than normal and beat more quickly. X-rays will show the heart to be enlarged or misshapen, and a tracing of the heart's electrical activity, an ECG, will also be abnormal. Sometimes, such a murmur may be detected for the first time when the puppy is checked by the vet for his first vaccination. Depending on the cause of the murmur, symptoms may not develop until later in life, if at all, particularly if the puppy seems otherwise perfectly normal. Some breeds, however, seem particularly affected by heart abnormalities. The Cavalier King Charles Spaniel is one in which almost fifty per cent of adults over five years of age are affected by heart murmurs.

Treatment The best treatment for congenital heart defects is surgical repair but this is only possible in certain types of defects in a few specialist veterinary centres. In most cases, severely restricting exercise and prescribing heart stimulants and diuretics may temporarily improve the situation. However, many affected puppies will die at an early age from heart failure.

CONGENITAL REGURGITATION AND VOMITING PROBLEMS

Regurgitation occurs when the puppy simply lowers his head and deposits undigested food on the floor without any muscular effort. Vomiting is a forceful expulsion of stomach contents by contraction of the stomach and abdominal muscles.

As most obstructions block the digestive tract only partially, symptoms usually start when the puppy is weaned on to solid food. Affected puppies are permanently hungry but underweight as they cannot keep food down.

Constriction of the Oesophagus

Regurgitation of food occurs when there is a partial or complete constriction of the oesophagus (gullet) so that solid food, instead of passing straight into the stomach, accumulates in the oesophagus causing it to distend. Vomiting usually occurs immediately after swallowing. In addition to being hungry and underweight, affected puppies often develop a cough because food overflows from the oesophagus into the trachea. This cough may develop into a fatal pneumonia.

The distended oesophagus is detected by an X-ray after a barium meal. There are two main causes of this condition:

Achalasia

Achalasia is caused by a thickening of a muscle, the cardiac sphincter, at the entrance to the stomach.

Treatment Surgery is not satisfactory. However, by giving liquid food in frequent small amounts from a raised feeding bowl, regurgitation can be eliminated in many

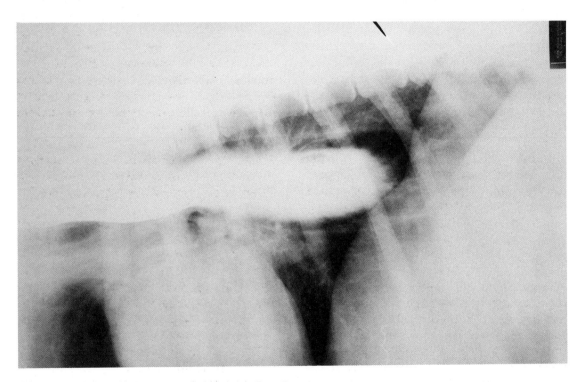

A barium meal X-ray shows up a case of achalasia in a Great Dane.

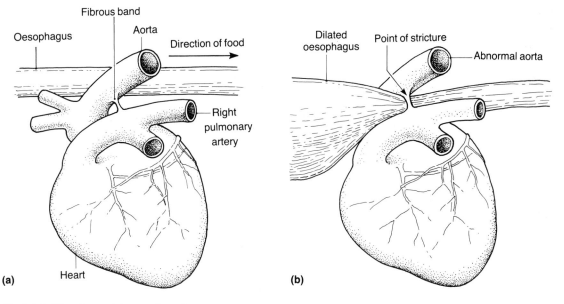

Fig 4 (a) View of normal heart and oesophagus
(b) Oesophageal stricture due to a developmental abnormality of the aorta

cases and the dog may improve in condition.

Persistent right aortic arch

An abnormality in the development of the large blood vessels where they leave the heart causes a ligament-like remnant of an artery to encircle and constrict the oesophagus.

Treatment Surgery is necessary through the chest wall to dissect away the offending blood vessel. Once the constriction is removed, the oesophageal function returns to normal and the regurgitation stops.

Pyloric Stenosis

This condition is caused by an overdevelopment of the muscle which regulates food outflow from the stomach, the pyloric sphincter. Persistent vomiting occurs, not immediately after swallowing as in the previous condition, but after a delay of one to two hours. An affected puppy is underweight and hungry, as insufficient food is retained. Diagnosis of pyloric stenosis is difficult even after a barium meal and X-ray, but modern techniques, involving fluoroscopy, are becoming more available and may make diagnosis easier. To establish a definite diagnosis it is often necessary to perform an abdominal operation to examine the pyloric sphincter.

Treatment A small but precise incision through the sphincter will relieve the constriction, and allow the stomach to empty normally.

INCONTINENCE

Many puppies have poor bladder control at the age of weaning and urinate at the least excitement. This usually settles down as the puppy grows but some bitch puppies will constantly drip urine for some time. One cause is an excessively short urethra, which is the tube from the bladder to the

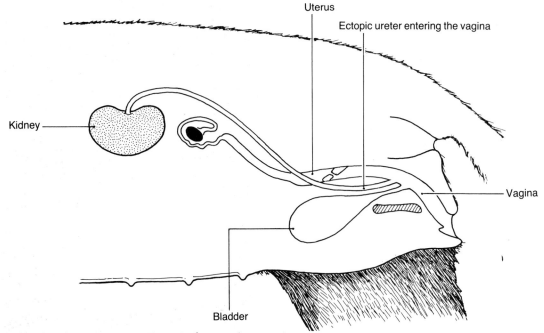

Fig 5 Bitch with ectopic ureter (see Figure 37 for normal anatomy)

vagina. As many of these incontinent bitches will improve after the first heat, surgical correction is delayed until this age in case it is not necessary.

Another cause of incontinence is a developmental defect of the ureter, a tiny tube conveying urine from the kidney to the bladder. In this defect, called an ectopic ureter, the ureter bypasses the bladder and enters directly into the vagina. Diagnosis is complicated and requires X-rays and the use of special radio-opaque dyes, injected into the urinary system.

Treatment Surgical correction of this defect consists of redirecting the ureter so that it enters the bladder at the correct site.

JUVENILE VAGINITIS

This occurs occasionally in bitch puppies when a reddish grey discharge from the vagina is seen. It rarely affects the puppy's

general health and nearly always ceases after the first heat period.

Treatment No treatment may be necessary but if the discharge is profuse, antibiotics may be helpful.

SKIN PROBLEMS

Many puppies of about twelve weeks of age, especially the short-coated breeds, may have white specks of dandruff throughout the coat. Provided the puppy is not itchy and has no lesions, thorough grooming or a wash with a veterinary shampoo may be all that is required. As the puppy grows, the condition usually settles down.

Sarcoptic Mange

This disease can affect all ages of dog but it is more common in the young puppy. It is caused by a parasitic mite which lives in the skin and causes intense irritation. The most commonly affected areas are the muzzle, ear flap, belly and legs. An affected puppy will scratch constantly which causes inflammation of the skin and hair loss. This damaged skin often becomes infected with bacteria. In severe cases, the skin becomes thickened, pigmented and scurfy. The puppy will lose weight and become very depressed.

The mite can be found by examining a scraping of the skin under a microscope. They are not easy to locate as they are not present in large numbers and several skin samples may be needed to find a single specimen.

Treatment The sarcoptic mite is killed with parasiticidal washes, but these must be repeated at regular intervals until the puppy stops scratching. In severe cases, antibiotics and sedatives may also be required.

As sarcoptic mange is very infectious, affected puppies must be isolated from other dogs. Any in-contact animals, bedding or kennelling should be washed in the parasiticide. This disease will cause transient irritation in people, especially children, causing very itchy little red spots (animal scabies), but it responds rapidly to treatment.

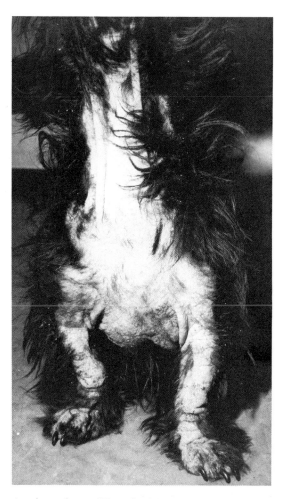

An advanced case of Demodectic Mange.

Demodectic Mange

This disease is less common than sarcoptic mange and is almost exclusively seen in puppies of three to nine months of age, especially in the short-coated breeds. The mite lives in the hair follicles and is thought to be present in most dogs in small numbers causing no symptoms. In some puppies, for reasons that are not clear, the mite starts to multiply causing, initially, patches of hair loss around the face and legs. In the early stages, there is no irritation and therefore the puppy does not scratch. As the disease progresses, the areas of hair loss increase, the damaged skin becomes infected and the puppy may now start to scratch. Severely infected dogs will be depressed and show extensive hair loss. The skin will be thickened, pigmented and greasy and it will have a very unpleasant smell. Demodectic mites are relatively easy to find on a skin scraping examined under the microscope.

Treatment Treatment, however, is not so easy. Any secondary bacterial infection must be treated with the appropriate antibiotic, identified by taking a swab, and the skin cleaned with a veterinary shampoo. A specific parasiticidal lotion is then applied to the bald areas, until the hair starts to regrow, which may take weeks or months. Despite intensive treatment, the outcome is not always successful.

Demodectic mange is acquired by the puppy congenitally from the dam and is not infectious to other dogs.

Pyoderma

At weaning time, many puppies have pustules on the hairless part of the belly. These spots usually cause no problems and disappear after a few weeks. In severe cases, antibiotic creams or tablets may be prescribed.

Juvenile Pyoderma (Head Gland Disease)

This is an uncommon but serious disease of young puppies between three and ten weeks of age. It usually affects just one puppy in the litter but, occasionally, the whole litter may become infected. The disease is caused by the Staphylococcus bacterium.

The owner will first notice that the puppy's head is developing swellings, especially around the eyelids, lips and under the jaw, but the puppy at this stage is only slightly unwell. The swellings will often develop into abscesses which may then appear elsewhere on the puppy's body. If the infection becomes extensive, the puppy will refuse food and quickly lose weight.

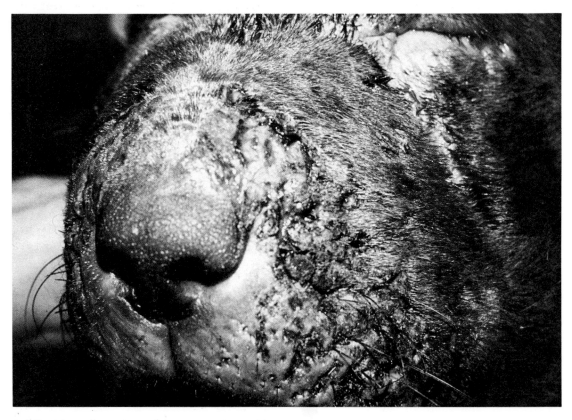

Bull Terrier puppy with juvenile pyoderma.

Treatment The discharging abscesses should be cleaned regularly with a warm, salt solution and the puppy should be isolated from his litter mates and mother. Antibiotics will be prescribed by the vet, often after laboratory testing to identify the correct drug.

Head gland disease can take several weeks to cure and the puppy may be left with a badly scarred face.

EAR MITES

These parasitic mites live in the ear canals of cats and dogs and are common in puppies. They are often first found by the vet at the time of vaccination. The mites initially cause an increase in wax secretion; but as they multiply, the irritation increases and the ear fills with wax. The puppy will shake his head or scratch at his ear. Many owners consider that the wax looks like dried blood.

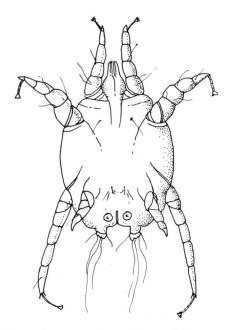

Fig 6 Ear mite (microscopic – greatly magnified)

Treatment The mites are readily seen through an auriscope and are easily killed with parasiticidal drops instilled into the ear. Treatment must be continued for six weeks or more to completely eliminate the infection, as the eggs laid in the ear by the mites are resistant to treatment. Mites spread rapidly to other dogs and cats and likely contacts should be treated at the same time.

DENTAL PROBLEMS

The milk teeth start to appear at about fourteen days of age. At four months of age, the permanent teeth begin to develop under the milk teeth, which they then push out as they grow. Under normal circumstances the milk teeth will have been totally replaced by the permanent teeth by the age of six months.

Occasionally permanent teeth, especially the canine and incisor teeth may erupt in the wrong place or in the wrong direction. Unfortunately, little can be done for misaligned teeth as most dogs will not tolerate a brace! If a tooth is grossly out of position, extraction may be necessary. Overcrowding of the molar teeth can occur in short-nosed dogs, leading to particles of food collecting between these teeth. This, in turn, leads to infection and to receding gums later in life.

Retention of the temporary teeth beyond six months of age is a common occurrence in the toy breeds and, in our experience, occurs most often in the Yorkshire Terrier. These retained teeth can cause two problems. Firstly, the developing permanent teeth are forced out of position and secondly, food can accumulate between the milk and permanent teeth causing gum disease. Temporary teeth that are still present after six months of age should be removed under an anaesthetic as soon as it becomes apparent that they will not be shed

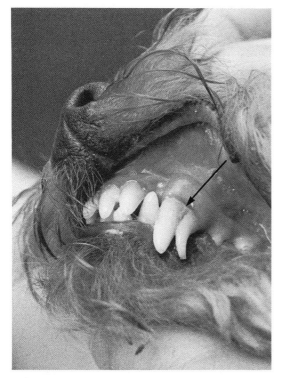

Plaque can be seen forming between the smaller retained temporary canine tooth and the larger permanent canine in this terrier.

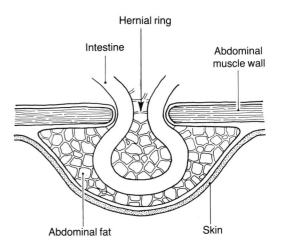

Fig 7 Diagrammatic representation of a hernia

normally. Canine and incisor teeth are again the ones most commonly implicated. When retained the root is often very long, at least the same length as the crown.

HERNIAS

A hernia is a hole or rupture in the body wall, through which loops of bowel or other abdominal organs can protrude. If this bowel or organ becomes trapped in the hernia and then swells due to constriction of its blood supply, the hernia is said to be strangulated. This then becomes an emergency.

Umbilical Hernia

The most common hernia seen in puppies is an umbilical hernia and occurs where the umbilical cord was attached to the puppy from the placenta. In most cases, only a small piece of abdominal fat protrudes and this often becomes sealed off so that the hernia cannot be reduced by finger pressure.

Treatment Treatment of small hernias may not be necessary, but if the hole is large enough for a loop of intestine to pass through, the defect must be repaired surgically. The ideal age for this, provided the puppy is otherwise healthy, is about five months of age.

Inguinal Hernia

Inguinal hernias occur in the groin but are very rare in the puppy. Surgical repair is necessary, again at about five months of age.

Scrotal Hernia

Scrotal hernias of male puppies occasionally occur and require surgical correction, at about four to five months of age. The first sign is usually an enlarged scrotum containing loops of bowel.

5 Common Infectious Diseases

DISTEMPER (HARD PAD)

Distemper is a highly infectious, frequently fatal virus disease which usually, but not always, affects dogs under one year of age. In large cities, where there is a high risk of unvaccinated dogs contacting each other, the disease is still frequently seen although widespread vaccination of dogs against distemper by responsible owners has reduced the incidence considerably. The virus is very fragile and is rapidly destroyed outside the body, so direct contact is the only method of spread.

The infection is normally contracted by inhalation of the virus from affected dogs, who shed the virus in cough droplets or in the discharges from the eyes and nostrils. Once inhaled, the virus divides rapidly in the tonsils and nearby lymph nodes. After a day or two, the virus appears in the blood stream, causing a mild temperature rise. It then begins to attack the epithelial cells of the body. These are the cells which line the surfaces of the body – skin, eyes, nose, bronchi of the lungs and the bowel. Signs of involvement of these structures usually do not develop until two weeks or so after the initial contact with an infected dog. This is called the incubation period. After approximately two more weeks, the virus will often attack the brain and other nerves, although the nervous symptoms may take several months or years to develop.

Clinical symptoms

Respiratory signs As distemper can vary from a very mild infection to a severe fatal one, so the symptoms vary and can mimic other diseases. Initially, the symptoms are those of a respiratory infection as the virus attacks the lining of the nose, throat and lungs. Affected dogs cough and begin to show a mild discharge from the eyes and nose. This usually progresses to a thick green or yellow purulent discharge. The eyes become very inflamed, appear reddened and the discharge from the nose dries in the nostrils making it difficult for the dog to breathe. Due to the effect of the virus on the lining of the trachea (windpipe) and the bronchi in the lungs, the dog will frequently cough – a whooping-cough-like noise – as he tries to clear his windpipe of discharge. This discharge will frequently be coughed up and swallowed although it is not uncommon for sputum to be coughed out.

Intestinal signs Shortly after this, the lining of the stomach and intestine can be affected resulting in vomiting and diarrhoea, sometimes with blood present. During this phase of the disease, the dog feels very miserable, has a raised temperature up to 40°C (104°F) is often off his food and spends most of the time just sleeping. His bouts of inactivity coincide with a fluctuating temperature which can vary from hour to hour or day to day. The respiratory and intestinal signs usually last about three weeks.

Skin signs In a generalised distemper infection, the virus next attacks the skin. The effects are particularly seen on the pads of the feet which become thickened and hard (hard pad). In a classic case, the dog can be heard tapping as he walks from the waiting room into the surgery on the hard floor. In addition, the normally cold, wet nose becomes dry and hard and this adds to the discomfort caused by the caking of the nostrils with discharge. As the affected dog cannot smell his food he will often not eat. In addition, blockage of the nostrils may mean the dog will have to breathe through his mouth.

At this stage, untreated cases will often develop pneumonia, due to a secondary infection with bacteria, and may die.

Nervous signs Some dogs, who survive the first stage, may then begin to show nervous symptoms. These usually develop some four weeks or so after the initial infection, but they may be delayed for many months in some cases. The symptoms are caused by the virus attacking the brain and they develop in three main ways, which may occur singly or in combination.

1 **Fits** Fits are the most common nervous symptom seen in distemper. A perfectly normal dog will suddenly develop a violent convulsion which will last from a few seconds to a few hours.

2 **Chorea** This is referred to as St Vitus's Dance. This peculiar twitch or jerk of one or more parts of the body can be most distressing for both the owner and the dog. It usually involves a limb or the head and is a repeated, rhythmical, reflex twitch which cannot be controlled. Once established, chorea does not usually subside.

3 **Paralysis** Usually affecting the hind quarters, this paralysis is seen as a gradual or sudden loss of use of the hind legs. Affected dogs have to pull themselves along by the front legs only.

Diagnosis In a classic case, there is little that distemper can be confused with. The nervous signs, following a respiratory infection in an unvaccinated dog, are considered diagnostic in practice.

There are, in fact, few diagnostic tests available for the live dog. In the early stages of the disease, your vet can gently take scrapings from the tonsils or lining of the lower eye lid. A laboratory may be able to detect the virus in these scrapings. More recently, a test has been developed which can detect distemper by analysing the urine of affected dogs. However, none of these tests is completely reliable. Even at post-mortem examination the virus cannot always be found in the tissue, although examination of the brain cells is the most reliable.

In young puppies, the distemper virus attacks the developing permanent teeth while they are still inside the gums. The enamel is affected, and when the teeth erupt at four to six months of age, many of them will be seen to be imperfect and show pits in the enamel. This is permanent but not painful or inconvenient to the dog. These so called 'distemper teeth' can be a useful aid to diagnosis after a suspected infection in a young puppy.

Treatment Like all virus infections, there is no specific cure for distemper. In the treatment of your dog, the vet will aim to control any secondary bacterial infection by using antibiotics. As the disease can last up to three weeks, careful nursing is essential.

In our experience, attention to making the patient comfortable and giving him a will to live is essential. His eyes should be bathed frequently with cotton wool soaked in warm sterile water, or saline, as often as is necessary to prevent the lids caking together with the discharge. They should be dried with a tissue immediately afterwards. The nose should be cleaned with petroleum jelly (not water as this will make it sore) and wiped away gently with tissues. If the patient can smell his food, he is more likely to eat it, so attention to the nose is important, as is the use of strong smelling, interesting foods.

Antibiotics may be injected, given in tablet or syrup form, and, in addition, as ointments or drops for the eyes. Their use may continue until the discharges from the eyes and nose have ceased and the cough has subsided. Your veterinary surgeon will decide.

Stomach sedatives may be used by your vet to control vomiting but light food such as fish, chicken, or scrambled egg helps. Kaolin suspension can be given to control diarrhoea. It is important, however, that the patient drinks a lot as fluid is necessary to counteract dehydration.

Cough medicines prescribed by your vet may be useful in controlling the coughing but do not be tempted to use a medical product for human use without checking with your vet first.

The nervous signs are difficult to treat. Fits may be controlled by anticonvulsant tablets or injections given by your vet. However, dogs which progress to this stage stand such a small chance of recovery that euthanasia is often recommended.

There are no medicines available that help control chorea or paralysis and the course of action recommended is dependent on the effect these signs are having on the dog. Occasionally, recovery will take place after several weeks or months but again, euthanasia may be the kindest course of action.

Vaccination It is far more sensible to prevent distemper than to try and cure it. If the dam (mother) of the puppies is immune to distemper, she will give them immunity in the form of antibodies in her colostrum. This is only temporary and fades by twelve weeks of age. Therefore, this is the best age for vaccination against distemper. However, if there is reason to suspect that the puppy was not given any immunity by the bitch, or if the puppy is thought to be in a high risk situation, then an additional vaccination can be given

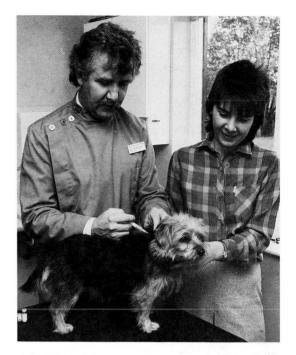

A healthy Norfolk Terrier has her annual vaccination.

earlier – but the twelve-week dose is still necessary. The puppy will not have developed sufficient immunity to protect him from distemper until about ten days after his vaccination so it is important to isolate him from other dogs for this period.

A vaccination booster each year against distemper is usually recommended throughout the dog's life.

INFECTIOUS CANINE HEPATITIS

This disease of the liver is caused by canine adenovirus type 1 (CAV–1). There is a type 2 (CAV–2) which is very similar, but causes a respiratory infection. The similarity between the two viruses is important when considering vaccination and this is discussed later in this chapter (*see* page 65).

Infectious canine hepatitis can occur in

both mild and severe forms. Usually young, unvaccinated dogs are affected.

Clinical symptoms Mildly affected patients are slightly off their food, appear somewhat dull and uninterested in life and have a raised temperature for a day or two. Recovery may be rapid and the vet will often diagnose the disease after the dog has recovered, due to the appearance of 'blue eye'. This is a bluish opacity in the cornea of one, or both, eyes and fortunately usually clears within two weeks.

In severe cases, the first sign may be a dog who is completely off his food, very dull and depressed and perhaps completely collapsed. Some dogs die suddenly, giving the owner no warning that anything is wrong. The temperature is usually over 40°C (104°F) to start with and the dog will show signs of acute discomfort in the abdomen, due to a painful swollen liver. The patient will be restless due to this abdominal pain. Vomiting will often occur and may contain specks of blood. The gums and inside lips may appear very pale, with small, widespread dots of haemorrhage for a few days. Jaundice may occur but this is not usual. Dogs suffering from this severe form of the disease are unlikely to recover.

The disease is spread by urine, faeces and saliva which all contain the virus. Indeed, recovered dogs can continue to excrete the virus for six months afterwards in the urine and thus spread the disease. In addition, the virus is very stable and can exist outside the body in the environment for as long as ten days, which means spread by indirect contact is possible.

The incubation period of the disease is usually about two weeks.

In very young puppies, infectious canine hepatitis is one of the causes of the fading puppy syndrome.

Diagnosis In mild cases the late appearance of 'blue eye' is usually the only method of

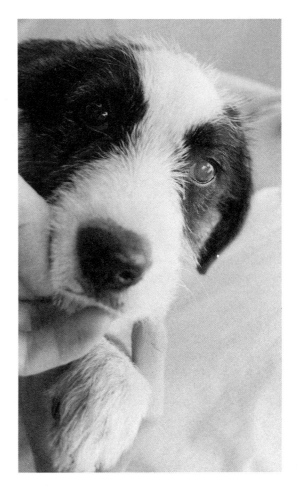

Blue eye affecting this puppy's left eye.

diagnosis. In severe cases, the symptoms are almost diagnostic and blood tests will help to confirm the disease. If the patient dies, a post-mortem and examination of liver tissue under a microscope will confirm the diagnosis.

Treatment There is no specific treatment for this disease. Any treatment given is aimed at the symptoms shown. Therefore, it is useful to give intravenous transfusions of a plasma substitute, glucose saline or even whole blood which helps counteract haemorrhage and shock, and to give drugs to stop vomiting. Antibiotics are often of no use, as the disease progresses so rapidly that there is no secondary bacterial infection.

Vaccination   Vaccination of young, susceptible puppies prevents development of the disease. This can be carried out using either CAV–1 or CAV–2 virus vaccines.

1 **CAV–1**   This vaccine is available either in live or dead forms.

The live vaccine will give a solid immunity when given to puppies of twelve weeks of age, or over. Occasionally, a side-effect is seen with this type of vaccine – 'blue eye' appears in one or both eyes about four weeks after the vaccination. Luckily, this usually disappears after a further few days.

The dead vaccine, given in two doses at eight to ten weeks and a second one at twelve weeks of age, gives a good immunity and is free from side-effects.

2 **CAV–2**   This vaccine is live and gives a good immunity after a single injection at twelve weeks of age or over. The side-effect of 'blue eye' does not occur with this vaccine. An added advantage is that protection is also given against the respiratory disease caused by the virus.

With both types of vaccine, a booster is usually recommended each year.

LEPTOSPIROSIS

Two separate forms of the organism Leptospira cause disease in the dog. *Leptospira canicola* causes acute kidney disease. *Leptospira icterohaemorrhagiae* causes an acute infection in the liver, often leading to jaundice.

In addition to causing severe and often fatal disease in the dog, both forms are infectious to humans. When diagnosing these diseases vets must also take into account the potential risks to the owner and all who handle the dog. This type of infection, transmissible between man and animals, is called a zoonosis.

Leptospira Canicola

Clinical symptoms   This disease is usually transmitted through infected urine which may be licked or inhaled by a susceptible dog. This was once a common disease and was known as 'Lamppost disease' for obvious reasons. It is in fact a disease mainly of town dogs, where urine stains are frequently investigated by other dogs. As the *Leptospira* organism is rapidly destroyed by sunlight and drying, dogs in sparsely populated countryside areas are much less at risk. The organisms invade the bloodstream for a week or so before attacking the kidney tissue. During this period, the dog may appear symptomless or show vague signs such as dullness and slight indifference to food.

After the incubation period the signs become much more severe with depression, total lack of interest in food, excess thirst and urination, vomiting and abdominal pain over the kidneys. If the kidneys are so severely affected that normal function ceases, then mouth ulcers and an unpleasant smell to the breath may develop. Death may follow, or the vet may advise euthanasia because of the low chance of recovery and the risk of spread of the disease to the owners.

Diagnosis   The clinical signs alone may be diagnostic in an unvaccinated town dog. Confirmation of the disease can be carried out by identifying the organism in blood or urine samples. If the patient dies, examination of the kidneys will usually confirm the diagnosis.

Treatment   The organism is susceptible to some antibiotics, notably the penicillins, oxytetracyclines and streptomycin, so treatment with any one of these will often result in a cure. In severe cases, intravenous fluid therapy with glucose saline is necessary. Anabolic steroids and vitamins may also help recovery.

Recovered dogs may be left with damaged kidneys and it is thought that this can lead to chronic kidney disease in the older dog.

Vaccination A combined vaccine against both *Leptospira canicola* and *Leptospira icterohaemorrhagiae* is available and has been in widespread use for several decades. This dead vaccine gives adequate protection against both diseases but only for about one year. Therefore, annual revaccination is necessary. Vaccination against leptospirosis forms part of the routine vaccination programme of puppies and is administered in two injections, two to four weeks apart, in combination with other vaccines starting at eight to twelve weeks of age. Widespread use of this vaccine has been responsible for the dramatic reduction in the incidence of this disease in recent years, which is now seen only in small numbers of unvaccinated town dogs.

Leptospira Icterohaemorrhagiae

Although this disease affecting the liver of the dog is very serious, widespread vaccination has reduced the number of cases seen to a very low level. This is mainly a country disease and rats frequently act as carriers to both dogs and man. The disease is transmitted through their urine.

Clinical symptoms The disease, as with *Leptospira canicola*, is spread by infected urine and enters the body via the mouth or nose. After entering the bloodstream, the organisms mainly attack the liver. The onset of illness is usually very sudden and very severe. Due to a raised temperature, the dog becomes very dull and depressed.

The eyes, gums, and skin turn yellow due to jaundice. Vomiting and diarrhoea, sometimes containing blood, may occur and the patient will often become very thirsty. Characteristic numerous small haemorrhages may appear in the gums and eyes, and severe conjunctivitis may develop. There is usually a rapid deterioration in the dog's condition over the first few days, although death can occur within a few hours of the first symptoms.

Diagnosis A diagnosis on the basis of symptoms is usually all that is necessary, although tests similar to those for *Leptospira canicola* can be used. If the patient dies, confirmation of diagnosis can be carried out at post-mortem using liver samples.

Treatment If diagnosed, or suspected early enough, antibiotic treatment may prevent the massive infection of the liver and thus prevent the severe disease from developing. Once the liver is affected to the degree that jaundice appears, treatment is usually ineffective. Bearing in mind the risk of infection to humans, and the discomfort suffered by the dog, euthanasia is often recommended.

Vaccination As with *Leptospira canicola*, the disease can be completely prevented by vaccination. The vaccinations for *Leptospira icterohaemorrhagiae* are given at exactly the same time and with the same vaccination as for *Leptospira canicola*.

CANINE PARVOVIRUS

The virus that causes this disease is very resistant to environmental changes and can live outside the body for well over a year. It is very similar to the feline enteritis virus and almost certainly developed from that virus.

In 1978 no one had heard of canine

parvovirus. Indeed, using blood samples in storage from before that time, it is possible to state that parvovirus did not exist before 1978. A change in the cat enteritis virus occurred and this new virus rapidly spread to all corners of the earth where it caused the disease of parvovirus. The dog population was totally susceptible. In general practice, vets began to suspect that there was a new problem because of unexpected deaths after signs of enteritis or heart disease. Our first cases were two Miniature Dachshunds from the same household. They both died.

Method of infection Infection occurs when the dog takes the virus into the mouth. In most cases, this occurs through direct contact with infected dogs or their faeces, which contain profuse amounts of the virus. However, as the virus can survive for long periods in the environment, infection is possible in two other important ways:

1 By the dog sniffing or investigating an area where infected faeces were passed months previously.
2 By the virus being brought into a safe area (house or garden, for example) on shoes or clothing.

These two factors are extremely important when attempting the elimination of disease from boarding or breeding kennels.

Heart Disease – Myocarditis

The virus attacks rapidly-dividing cells. In a susceptible young puppy, from one to three weeks old, the heart muscle is developing very rapidly and the virus attacks and damages these heart cells. Most puppies will die by eight weeks of age although a small number may die when older. Some survive but they have a weakened heart.

This form of the disease was commonly seen at the start of the outbreak in 1978/79 but as the dog population became resistant, puppies were given antibodies by their mothers and so had protection at this early stage. Parvovirus myocarditis is now extremely rare and we have not seen a case since 1980 in our practice.

Parvovirus Enteritis

By the time the maternal antibodies are fading, from weaning onwards, the lining cells of the intestine are multiplying rapidly and the virus now attacks these cells. Any age of dog is susceptible but infection is commonest in puppies. In the twelve-week age group, the death rate is about ten per cent. The stress of change of ownership at this age can sometimes precipitate the disease, while puppies remaining with the breeder may show no symptoms.

Clinical symptoms Usually signs appear suddenly with vomiting, depression and anorexia. The vomiting can be difficult to stop and the dog can rapidly become dehydrated and lose much weight. This is made worse by the appearance of diarrhoea, usually within about twenty-four hours. The diarrhoea is very watery, often with blood, and has a characteristic foul smell. Symptoms, however, are very variable and the faeces may range from profusely haemorrhagic to merely a little soft. The dog's temperature may or may not be raised. Unless treated, death from dehydration can occur rapidly within two or three days.

Diagnosis Clinical symptoms can be very useful to suspect the disease and initiate treatment, but are not diagnostic.
The virus can usually be detected in the faeces of an affected dog by a laboratory. Blood can be tested for the presence of parvovirus antibodies and the level of these will confirm the infection. If the dog dies,

parvovirus can be confirmed by micro-scopic examination of the bowel or heart muscle.

Treatment As death is usually due to dehydration, prompt and proper replacement of the fluid and electrolyte loss is essential. A fluid called Hartman's solution is given by drip feed into the vein and for this reason your vet will hospitalise your dog. Where the dog is very shocked, plasma substitutes or even whole blood may have to be given.

In addition, antibiotics are also usually given to prevent secondary bacterial infection from making the situation worse. Prompt treatment can lead to a rapid recovery, especially in adult dogs, but some cases, for instance where the bowel lining is severely affected, take longer. Attention to diet in these dogs is very important. Low bulk, light food such as fish, chicken, rice, and scrambled egg is ideal. Some dogs are left with a damaged digestive system.

Prevention

Vaccination The history of parvovirus vaccination is interesting. When the disease first appeared in 1978, there was no specific vaccine available. Vets had to turn to the cat enteritis vaccines which gave some protection to dogs against the similar virus. We first used the dead cat vaccines and then the live ones to achieve a better result. Soon vaccines were developed from the canine parvovirus itself and these give nearly a one hundred per cent protection.

Most adult dogs are now immune to the disease by either previous exposure or vaccination, so puppies receive maternal antibodies from their dam. In most cases, these antibodies will give protection for up to eight weeks and sometimes up to eighteen weeks of age, but they will also interfere with vaccination. Thus, puppies vaccinated before this age may require a further vaccination against parvovirus at about twenty weeks of age, to ensure adequate immunity.

Recently a live vaccine has been developed which, it is claimed, gives complete protection at twelve weeks of age.

In practice, parvovirus vaccination is given in combination with distemper, hepatitis and leptospirosis vaccination from eight weeks of age onwards, and many vets give an additional parvovirus vaccination at sixteen to twenty weeks of age. Annual boosters are recommended.

Infected premises It is very difficult to eradicate the disease from infected premises such as kennels, where many dogs are present. Vaccination of puppies may fail because of the high level of maternal antibodies which may then wane before the next vaccine is given, leading to disease. A plan of action must be undertaken, as follows.

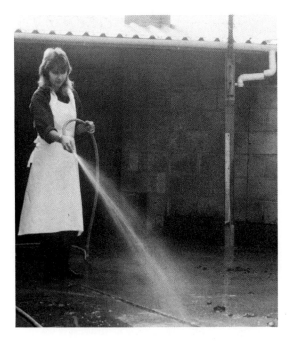

Thorough mechanical cleaning with water is essential prior to disinfection.

1 Vaccination of puppies from six weeks of age and then every two weeks.
2 Thorough mechanical cleaning of the premises using pressure hosing, if possible.
3 Disinfection of the cleaned premises. Parvovirus is very resistant to disinfection and is only killed by hypochlorite (bleach) or formalin, which can be purchased commercially. Fumigation by formalin may help.
4 Compartmentalisation of the kennels so that puppies can be reared in isolated batches.
5 Personal hygiene and attention to detail by the staff. For example, boots should be disinfected after entering each isolation kennel, hands thoroughly washed and separate overalls worn in each kennel.

KENNEL COUGH

As the name implies, this is a very infectious respiratory infection occurring especially in dogs kept in kennels. It occurs most frequently in kennels with a changing population, such as a boarding kennel or stray dogs' home, where newly introduced dogs either bring in the infection or acquire it from affected inmates. A constant cycle of infection can, therefore, develop.

Any infectious cough which affects dogs will be called 'kennel cough' as this name covers a multitude of causes. These range from a sore throat, as a result of excess barking, to several specific infections. The main causes are as follows.

Bordetella bronchiseptica is a bacterial infection which affects the trachea and lungs. It can be a primary infection or follow another virus infection.
Canine adenovirus can cause kennel cough.
Canine herpesvirus is especially associated with the disease in young puppies.
Canine parainfluenza virus is seen in Great Britain where it complicates other respiratory infections, but is known to be a main cause of kennel cough in the USA.

Clinical symptoms Although the disease can, and does, occur in dogs which have not been in kennels, the symptoms are most frequently seen in dogs in kennels or within five to ten days of being kennelled. The dog develops a cough which may be mild to start with but rapidly becomes severe. Often the owner is convinced that the dog has 'something stuck in his throat'. Coughing can become paroxysmal or may just be mild and intermittent. Excitement, such as responding to the door bell or exercise, usually brings on a bout of coughing.

In most cases, this mild or severe cough is the only symptom. Dogs remain bright and alert, and their appetite remains good. Occasionally, a purulent discharge from the nose and eyes may develop.

Diagnosis The occurrence of a cough shortly after kennelling is usually considered diagnostic. During the clinical examination, the vet may be able to stimulate the cough reflex in affected cases by gently pressing on the trachea.

Treatment Antibiotics are usually prescribed by the vet because *Bordetella* bacteria are frequently involved either as a primary or secondary infection.

Rest is very important in the treatment of this disease. We have known cases last for months where the owner would not, or could not, rest his dog whereas other cases have cleared up in a matter of days with the correct nursing. The dog should not be allowed to become chilled and he should be kept dry and warm. His food should be soft so it can be easily swallowed.

Proprietary cough medicines can help to depress the cough but if the trachea becomes affected, by an accumulation of infected mucus, the cough reflex is essential to expel this.

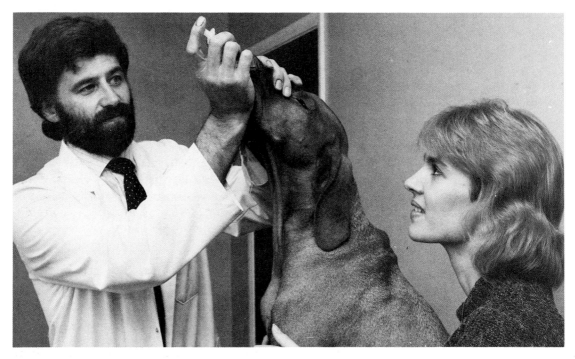

A Hungarian Viszla has her Kennel Cough vaccination.

Very occasionally pneumonia will follow, especially in debilitated or old dogs, and death can occur.

Prevention In Great Britain and the USA the main cause of kennel cough, *Bordetella*, can be prevented by vaccination. This vaccine, given in droplet form into the nostrils of the dog, should be administered about two weeks before kennelling. It is generally tolerated well and gives a good immunity for about six months. Vaccination against canine *parainfluenza* virus and canine *adenovirus* can be included in the dog's routine vaccine course but these two are considered less important in Great Britain than *Bordetella*.

RABIES

Rabies is a virus disease which affects the central nervous system. Many species are affected throughout the world. The main hosts are the dog, cat, fox, vampire bat, skunk and mongoose.

Rabies is present in the continents of Europe, America, India and Asia but not Australia. However, within these continents certain countries are free of rabies – notably Great Britain and Ireland, Portugal, some Scandinavian countries and Japan. France has many cases each year, especially in the fox population. Rabies is under control in the USA, but in certain areas there are some species of animals which are carriers of the disease, mainly bats, skunks, raccoons and foxes.

Spread of the disease The virus is spread by a susceptible animal being bitten by an infected animal. It cannot penetrate intact skin but can gain entry through a pre-existing cut. The virus enters a nerve ending in the skin and travels from here up the nerve to the spinal cord; then it travels slowly up to the brain. So far the animal is symptomless and the original wound will have healed. Once in the brain, the virus spreads down the nerves to the salivary glands and into the saliva in the mouth. It then spreads to another animal when this saliva is introduced through a bite.

Clinical symptoms As the virus travels along the nerves, the length of the incubation period is determined by the size of the dog and the site of the bite. It is usually between ten days and four months. A Jack Russell Terrier bitten on the neck will develop rabies much sooner than a Great Dane bitten on the end of his tail.

The first sign that a dog has rabies is a change in his temperament. Friendly dogs become suspicious or aggressive, while aggressive nervous dogs may become friendly. The temperature is raised. From this initial phase, rabies usually develops into one of two types:

1 **Furious rabies** The dog becomes more excitable, restless and develops an odd behaviour pattern. He may snap at imaginary objects and often has a depraved appetite, chewing and swallowing unusual objects, such as wood and stones. He becomes aggressive and chews fiercely at his lead if confined or attacks people or other animals. He may wander for miles and so the potential for spread is tremendous. An affected dog will then become weaker as paralysis sets in, will have difficulty swallowing and become progressively more comatose until death occurs.

2 **Dumb rabies** This is the commoner form and is more difficult to diagnose. The dog just becomes duller as paralysis sets in, and coma and death follow.

In both forms, death usually occurs within five days of the start of the classic symptoms. Affected dogs should not be handled or euthanased but should be confined and the case reported to the Ministry of Agriculture or health authorities of that country. Any in-contact dogs or cats should also be isolated until a diagnosis has been established.

Diagnosis In Great Britain, the above signs in a dog in quarantine would be sufficient to isolate the dog. Food and water are pushed through the bars but no one is allowed to be in contact with the dog. If death ensues, post-mortem examination of the brain will establish a diagnosis.

Prevention

Quarantine As rabies is always fatal once a human, dog or any other animal becomes infected, any dog entering from abroad is vaccinated and placed in quarantine for six months. This isolation has proved totally successful at keeping rabies out and Great Britain has been free of rabies since 1908.

Vaccination This gives a high degree of protection against rabies, but not one hundred per cent, so quarantine is a better way of keeping an island country like Great Britain free of rabies. Once a country is affected by the disease, however, vaccination is essential. In addition, a reduction in the number of strays, and a reduction in susceptible wildlife (in Great Britain and Europe this is the fox) is essential. To have any effect against rabies, at least seventy per cent of the dog population must be vaccinated.

Rabies in man Safe vaccines are now available and people in high-risk situations can be protected. This applies both to people bitten abroad or people working in Great Britain in situations where they may be exposed to rabies – for example, in quarantine kennels or vets working in channel port towns.

6 The Digestive System

The digestive system is composed of the mouth, throat or pharynx, gullet or oesophagus, stomach, intestines, liver and pancreas. Food is required by all animals for energy, growth and maintenance of body tissues, and the function of the digestive system is to provide this food in a form that the body can use. Food is taken into the body through the mouth, where it is chewed and swallowed. It is then broken down in the stomach and intestines by enzymes which are produced by the body in the salivary glands, stomach, pancreas and intestines. These enzymes attack the food and break it down into very small particles, such as glucose, which can be absorbed through the intestinal wall. Waste matter is evacuated via the rectum.

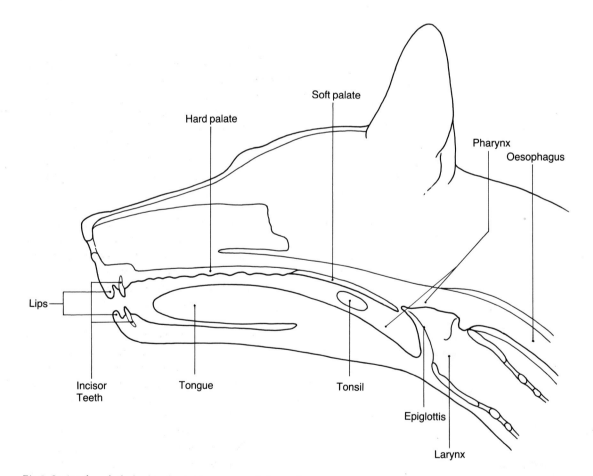

Fig 8 Section through the head to show main structures of the mouth

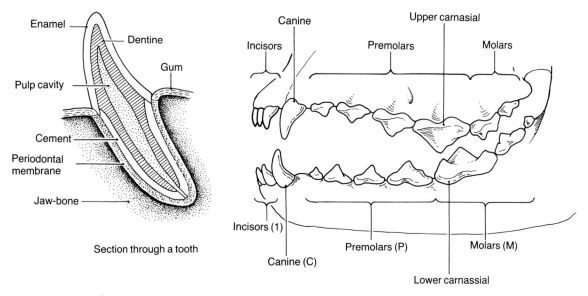

Fig 9 *Arrangement of teeth in the adult dog*

NORMAL STRUCTURE AND FUNCTION

The mouth contains the teeth, tongue and tonsils and is separated from the nasal chambers by the hard and soft palate. The main function of the mouth is to take in food and break it down into pieces which can be swallowed. A dog has twenty-eight milk teeth as a puppy and forty-two permanent teeth as an adult. Several salivary glands, the biggest being the parotid salivary gland, discharge saliva into the mouth and this lubricates the food and starts the process of digestion. The mouth is also used for breathing, when the dog is at full exercise, and is also involved in heat loss through panting.

Between the mouth and entrances to the oesophagus and larynx is the pharynx which both conducts air from the nose to the larynx and also starts the process of swallowing. The oesophagus is a straight muscular tube which passes from the pharynx, through the chest to the stomach. It has only one function, to convey food to the stomach.

The stomach is a muscular sac which stores and mixes the food and then continues the process of digestion with acid and enzymes produced by its lining. Food passes from the stomach through a muscular ring, the pylorus, into the small intestine. The small intestine is a long convoluted tube in which the food is finally broken down into its components which are then absorbed through the intestinal wall. The liver produces bile salts and the pancreas produces enzymes both of which are secreted through small ducts into the small intestine just below the pylorus.

Where the small intestine joins the large intestine there is a small sac-like structure called the caecum, which is the equivalent organ to the appendix in man. Inflammation of the caecum (appendicitis) is extremely rare in the dog. The first part of the large intestine is called the colon and here some food is absorbed but, more importantly, water is removed to produce dry faeces, or stools. Faeces, which consist of undigested food and gut bacteria, are stored in the last part of the large intestine, the rectum. The large intestine produces mucus which helps

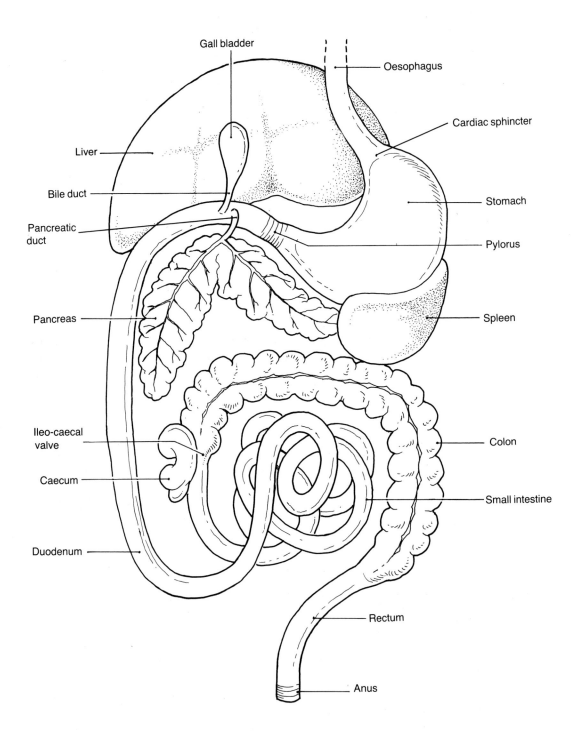

Fig 10 Diagram of the digestive system

in the evacuation of the faeces. The exit to the rectum is controlled by a strong muscular ring, the anus.

The part of the body which contains the stomach, intestines, liver and pancreas along with the kidneys, bladder and uterus is known as the abdomen. The inner walls of the abdomen and all its organs are covered by a shiny tissue, the peritoneum, which allows free movement of the organs within the abdomen.

DISEASES OF THE MOUTH AND PHARYNX

Inflammation of the Mouth

This can be caused by infection, injuries, the ingestion of toxic substances such as acids, or can be part of a generalised disease, such as kidney failure. The lining of the mouth becomes inflamed and, in severe cases, there will be ulceration of the tongue and palate causing the dog to salivate excessively and to refuse his food.

Treatment The condition is treated with antibiotics, and the dog is fed with soft foods. Concurrent diseases must also be treated.

Pharyngitis (Sore Throat)

This is a fairly common condition and often the symptoms can be mistaken for an obstruction of the throat. The pharynx is inflamed and may be ulcerated, causing the dog to gulp or retch. He will be reluctant to eat and may be depressed due to a raised temperature. Pharyngitis is frequently associated with the kennel cough syndrome.

Treatment Pharyngitis usually responds quickly to treatment with antibiotics.

Tonsillitis

This is a common condition in young dogs and produces symptoms similar to pharyngitis, but there may also be a soft cough. Tonsillitis may be a recurring problem and, occasionally, the tonsils may become so large that they cause obstruction of the pharynx. They are responsible for mopping up infection from the pharynx and so many diseases of the nose and mouth result in enlarged tonsils.

Treatment Early cases of tonsillitis usually respond to treatment with antibiotics but in severe cases surgical removal (tonsillectomy) is the treatment chosen.

Foreign Bodies

The mouth is often injured by foreign objects because the dog uses his mouth for catching and carrying objects and also for crunching bones.

Bones

Small pieces of bone can become wedged between the teeth. The dog will suddenly start to paw at his mouth, he will often be unable to close his jaws and there will be excessive salivation. The small piece of bone is easily removed, but in large or very distressed dogs this may require a general anaesthetic.

Sticks

By attempting to catch bouncing sticks, dogs frequently impale themselves and this can cause horrific injuries. The point of the stick may penetrate several inches into the soft tissues of the tongue, pharynx or soft palate. The dog will cry at the time of injury and he may not be able to close his mouth. The saliva will be blood-tinged and there may also be severe haemorrhage. The dog will subsequently refuse food.

Treatment These wounds must be thoroughly cleansed under a general anaesthetic, to remove any splinters of wood and infection. If large, the wound will be sutured with dissolving sutures, and antibiotics may be prescribed by your vet. The dog should be fed on soft food for a few days. These wounds heal quickly but abscess formation may occur even after several weeks, especially if any small splinters of wood remain in the wound.

Balls

Small rubber balls can also cause a serious problem as they may be accidentally swallowed and lodge in the pharynx, where they completely obstruct the airway. Death from asphyxiation can occur quickly.

Treatment (*See also* Chapter 18, page 221.) As the ball is smooth and covered in saliva it cannot readily be grasped and pulled out through the mouth. However, by pushing on the lower side of the neck, just behind the jaws, the ball can often be pushed out. If this proves impossible, take the dog immediately to the nearest vet.

Fish-Hooks

These can become caught in the mouth, usually penetrating through the lips. The vet will often remove the hook under a general anaesthetic. (*See also* Chapter 18, page 222.)

Salivary Gland Diseases

Infection

Infection produces a hot, painful and enlarged salivary gland which will make the dog unwilling to open his mouth to eat. Treatment usually involves antibiotics but if an abscess forms it may require lancing.

Salivary Gland Cysts

Salivary cysts are not uncommon and occur as painless swellings under the tongue or neck. The cyst is full of saliva from a ruptured salivary duct and if it is left untreated, it may become fairly large. In a Dachshund, for example, the cyst may be as large as an orange. If the cyst occurs under the tongue, the dog may have difficulty in eating.

Treatment There is no medical treatment and so the offending salivary gland and cyst must be removed surgically.

Tumours

The mouth is a common site for tumours. Most tumours are very malignant, grow quickly and readily spread to other organs. The most common sites of tumour growth are the gum margins and tonsils. Often the first sign is an increase in salivation, which may be blood-tinged. The dog may find it difficult to eat or swallow and often has an unpleasant smell on his breath.

Treatment Treatment is difficult because the tumour will usually have already invaded the hard tissues of the mouth, such as the jaw bone or hard palate. Cryosurgery (the killing of tissue by freezing) is often very successful if the tumour is detected early. Far more radical surgery, such as the removal of a portion of the jaw-bone, is possible provided there is no evidence of tumour spread to other organs.

Epulis

Small, hard nodules, called epuli are common on the gum margins, especially in Boxers. They are not malignant and usually cause no problem unless they grow between the teeth, or become so large the dog chews on them.

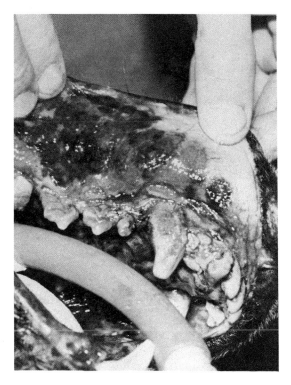

Severe plaque and periodontal disease. The dog is anaesthetised and the endotracheal anaesthetic tube can be seen.

Gingival Hyperplasia

This is an overgrowth of the gum margins, causing the teeth to become buried below the gum. It is common in Boxers, and is very similar to epulis formation but much more extensive.

Treatment In severe cases, it is necessary to cut the gum back to its original level using thermocautery.

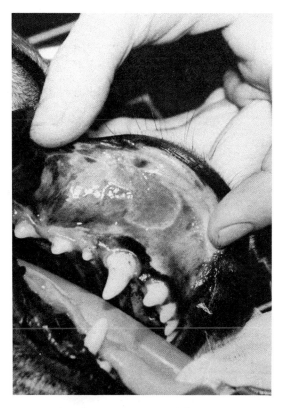

The same dog after the teeth were scaled.

DENTAL PROBLEMS

Dental Caries

Dental caries (commonly known as tooth decay) is far less of a problem in dogs than in people. It can, however, occasionally occur in the flat molar teeth at the back of the jaw where, surprisingly, it often appears to cause little discomfort. By the time the vet finds the caried tooth, the cavity may be quite large and the tooth may have to be extracted. Small cavities can be drilled out and filled.

Periodontal Disease

Periodontal disease of the gum around the tooth, however, is very common in the dog especially in the smaller breeds, because dental plaque readily forms on the teeth.

Treatment Surgical removal is normally recommended, usually involving thermocautery.

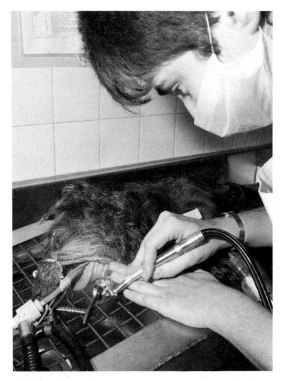

A veterinary nurse scales a patient's teeth with an ultrasonic dental scaler.

Plaque is a hard deposit composed of minerals and dead bacteria which slowly accumulates on the teeth, starting at the gum margin. Dental plaque irritates the gums causing inflammation, known as gingivitis. As the gingivitis causes gum recession the tooth roots become exposed. Infection can then enter the tooth socket causing further inflammation, loosening and loss of the tooth. Dogs with advanced gingivitis have an appalling mouth odour. Surprisingly, despite the most advanced dental disease, most dogs will continue to eat but they are much healthier and happier after dental treatment.

Prevention Only prevention of plaque formation will avoid the above sequence of events. The dog should be provided with hard objects to chew such as large raw marrow bones, chews, large hard biscuits, raw carrots, or dental toys. Unfortunately, the smaller breeds are usually fussy eaters

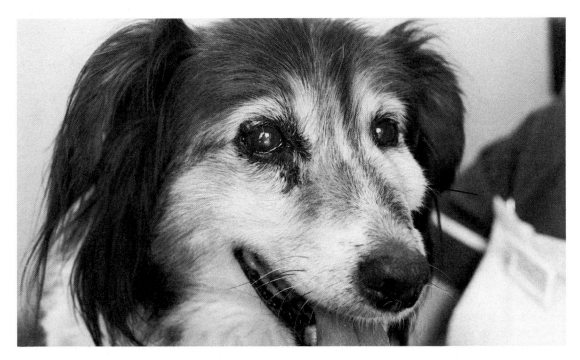

The swelling below the left eye is a malar abscess.

and will often only eat meat or soft food. Here the owner can help by regularly brushing their teeth but this is only possible in good tempered dogs. Regular removal of dental plaque under general anaesthesia is routinely carried out by vets and the proportion of dental cases in a normal day's work is quite high. Ultrasonic scalers are now commonplace in veterinary surgeries and the regular, gentle scaling and polishing of dogs' teeth results in a higher proportion of patients retaining their teeth into old age. Some dogs may never need to have their teeth scaled, while others may require scaling as often as every six months.

Treatment If periodontal disease is advanced, any loose teeth must be extracted and a course of antibiotics considered. Many dogs lose their teeth unnecessarily, as their owners have been unaware of the need for regular dental care.

Teeth may become broken through accidents, fights or by chewing very hard objects such as stones. The canines and upper carnassials (the large cutting teeth) are the teeth usually affected. Treatment of these fractures depends on their severity and position. Some small fractures can be ignored provided the pulp cavity has not been exposed. If the fracture is severe and irreparable, the vet may remove the affected tooth. However, in cases where a small chip is involved and the pulp cavity is exposed, your vet, if unable to operate himself, may enlist the help of a willing dentist to carry out root treatment and repair the defects. We have worked with a local dentist to fill various teeth and to repair fractured canine teeth with new crowns. This can give a very satisfactory, functional and cosmetic result.

An undetected fracture can lead to the formation of a root abscess which is usually first noticed when the dog refuses his food and has a painful swelling below the eye. If left untreated, this abscess may rupture and discharge down the cheek. The damaged tooth must be removed under a general anaesthetic, the abscess drained and antibiotic treatment instigated. This condition is referred to as a malar abscess, as the abscess discharges through the malar bone of the cheek.

DISEASES OF THE OESOPHAGUS

Obstruction

Blockage of the oesophagus can be caused by small bones such as chop bones. The dog is often very uncomfortable and off his food. Any food eaten will be regurgitated almost immediately. The foreign body can usually be seen on an X-ray, or by looking down the oesophagus with an oesophagoscope.

Treatment These foreign bodies must be removed as soon as possible before the oesophageal wall is seriously damaged. Sometimes, the object can be retrieved through the mouth with long forceps or it can be gently pushed into the stomach. Firmly embedded foreign bodies must be removed surgically by open chest surgery.

Achalasia

See Chapter 4, page 54.

DISEASES OF THE STOMACH AND INTESTINE

In many diseases of the stomach and intestine it is necessary to empty the bowel of food to prevent further irritation to its lining. This is achieved by withholding food for twenty-four hours but fluid intake must be encouraged. The bowel is then gently returned to normal by feeding a highly digestible low-fibre diet, such as boiled fish or chicken, boiled white rice, cottage cheese or cooked eggs, for three days. The dog's normal diet is then slowly introduced over the next three days. In the rest of this chapter this will be referred to as *withholding food and then feeding a light diet*.

Vomiting

Gastritis (Inflammation of the stomach)

Inflammation and ulceration of the stomach lining can be caused by infection, or by eating unsuitable food. The dog is depressed, may be off his food and repeatedly vomits either food or stomach fluid which can be bloodstained.

Treatment In mild cases, treatment simply consists of withholding food for twenty-four hours and then feeding a light diet. In severe cases, antibiotics and gastric sedatives may be necessary.

Foreign bodies

Foreign bodies, such as a stone or small ball, can block the pylorus or intestine. Complete blockage of the intestine is a very serious condition. The dog will become ill very quickly, and vomit frequently and persistently. His vomit will at first be yellow or white but, gradually, it will become brown and foul smelling. The dog will not eat or defaecate and there will be severe abdominal pain. The vet may be able to feel the obstruction through the body wall but an X-ray of the abdomen may be required to confirm the diagnosis.

Sometimes a foreign body, such as a handkerchief or plastic bag, will produce a partial obstruction. The symptoms will be similar to those described in the previous paragraph but they will not be so severe and the dog may pass some faeces. This type of foreign body may take several days to pass through the intestine. If it suddenly stops moving, there will be a marked

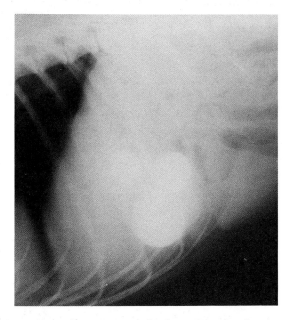

The four golf balls that this Labrador swallowed can be seen in the stomach on this X-ray.

deterioration in the dog's condition and emergency surgery will be required.

Treatment When an intestinal obstruction due to a foreign body has been diagnosed, the object is surgically removed as soon as possible. If the dog has become dehydrated he may require intravenous fluid therapy.

Intussusception

This condition is mainly seen in puppies during, or following, a bout of diarrhoea. The excess bowel contractions lead to a length of intestine becoming telescoped into the following section and this causes a blockage. The puppy will start to vomit and this will often contain blood. After a while, the diarrhoea will cease but the vomiting will continue and the puppy will become depressed and refuse food. The vet can often diagnose an intussusception by palpation through the body wall when a painful sausage-shaped swelling can be felt.

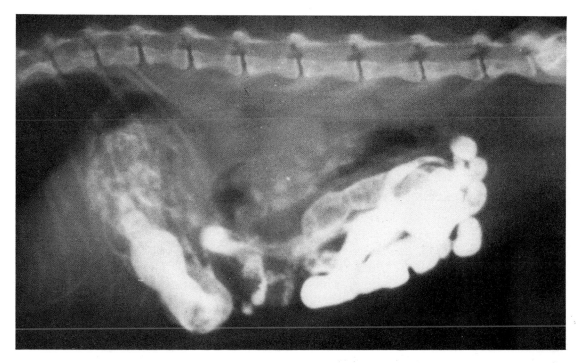

The stomach and intestines are outlined by barium on this X-ray.

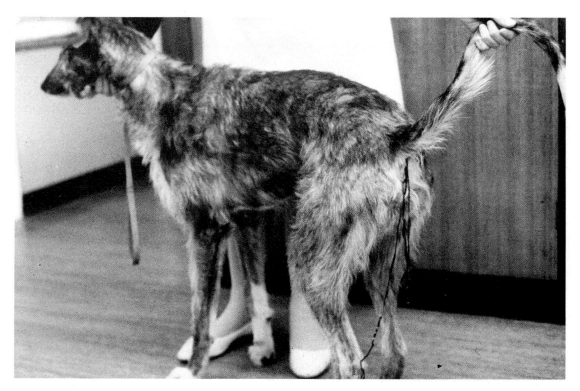

This Deerhound swallowed a cassette tape.

Treatment An emergency operation is required to reduce the intussusception. If the condition has been diagnosed at a very early stage, the telescoped portion can be gently manipulated out of the normal intestine. However, any delay may cause one portion of intestine to adhere to the other and it will be necessary to remove the damaged section by an operation called an enterectomy.

Tumours

Tumours of the stomach occasionally occur in the older animal and lead to an increasing frequency of vomiting which becomes bloodstained as the tumour grows. These tumours are painful so the dog will be depressed, have a poor appetite and show a gradual weight loss. Diagnosis is not always straightforward. Some tumours may be visible on an X-ray but others can only be diagnosed by an exploratory operation to examine the stomach.

Localised tumours of the intestine are fairly uncommon and in the early stages they cause no symptoms. It is only when they are large enough to obstruct the bowel that symptoms of intestinal obstruction occur – persistent vomiting (often of a brown colour) and absence of faeces. These tumours can be diagnosed on an X-ray after giving the dog a barium meal.

Treatment Unfortunately, stomach tumours are usually malignant and once diagnosed, euthanasia is the treatment of choice. Small bowel tumours can be removed surgically, provided there is no evidence of spread to other organs.

Gastric Dilatation and Torsion

This is a very serious condition in the older, larger dog, and is included in this section because, although no vomit is produced, the dog persistently tries to be sick.

In gastric dilatation, the stomach suddenly fills with gas shortly after a meal. The dog's abdomen becomes grossly distended and the increased abdominal pressure impairs respiration. The dog becomes depressed very quickly and can die within hours. The dilated stomach can become unstable and, in some cases, will actually twist within the abdomen to produce gastric torsion. This is more serious than gastric dilatation as the blood supply to the stomach is greatly reduced and both the entrance and exit to the stomach are occluded by the twist.

Treatment Gastric torsion and dilatation are genuine emergencies and the excess gas must be released from the stomach as quickly as possible. In gastric dilatation, this release of gas can be achieved by passing a tube down the oesophagus into the stomach, either in the conscious or anaesthetised dog. The stomach is then washed out through this tube. In gastric torsion, the tube cannot be passed into the stomach to release the gas, so a large hypodermic needle is inserted by the vet through the skin into the stomach. Following this release of pressure in the abdomen, which allows the dog to breathe more easily, an operation is necessary to return the stomach to its normal position. The dog will be in surgical shock and will require intravenous fluid therapy and intensive care. Recovery is by no means certain but, the quicker he is taken to the surgery, the better are his chances of survival.

Gastric dilatation can recur and any affected dogs should subsequently be fed several small meals a day, and never exercised within one hour of feeding.

Diarrhoea

Enteritis

Enteritis is the inflammation of the small intestine and can be caused by specific infections such as parvovirus, a heavy worm burden, food poisoning or unsuitable food. Enteritis is very common in dogs because of their natural scavenging habits.

The symptoms can vary enormously. In mild cases, the dog is perfectly normal, except for softish faeces. At the other extreme, the dog will be depressed, off his food and have frequent watery, blood-tinged diarrhoea. A dog which is not drinking and has severe diarrhoea can become dehydrated very quickly.

Treatment In mild cases, withholding solid food for twenty-four hours while ensuring an adequate supply of water may be the only treatment necessary. In more severe cases, in addition to withholding food, antibiotics or intestinal sedatives and oral fluid therapy may be required. In the severely dehydrated patient, fluid replacement by intravenous fluid therapy must be instigated as soon as possible; antibiotics may also be needed. Once the diarrhoea is under control, a light diet should be fed for several days.

Colitis

This is the inflammation of the large bowel or colon and usually produces a less severe diarrhoea than enteritis. The faeces tend to be soft rather than watery and there are often spots of blood and an increased amount of mucus. The dog appears to be healthy in all other respects.

Treatment Mild cases of colitis may respond to dietary management alone, along similar lines to treatment of enteritis, but more severe cases may require antibiotics and/or anti-inflammatory drugs. A sulphonamide drug called Salazopyrin is particularly useful in certain types of colitis.

Dietary Diarrhoeas

Any dog changing from one type of food to another may develop a mild diarrhoea. This seems to occur in puppies at the time of their first change of owner. These cases respond to dietary treatment; food should be withheld for twenty-four hours, followed by a low-fibre diet and a gradual introduction of the new diet over the next few days.

The large breeds of dog seem more likely to suffer from mild diarrhoea of dietary origin. The dogs are normally healthy, do not lose weight but they have persistent soft stools. In such cases, it is necessary to keep trying different diets until the most suitable one is found. It may be that dehydrated food or tinned food containing more roughage is ideal.

Malabsorption

This is an uncommon condition in which the intestinal wall is diseased and has a decreased ability to absorb digested food. Affected dogs have a ravenous appetite, lose weight and produce soft bulky faeces. For diagnosis of this condition, laboratory testing of blood and faeces and sometimes an intestinal biopsy are necessary.

Treatment Management of malabsorption is difficult and often unsatisfactory. Highly digestible food must be fed, such as rice, pasta and cottage cheese. Alternatively specially formulated prescription diets are available from your vet. Treatment with anti-inflammatory drugs and the addition of vitamin B12 and folic acid to the diet may help the absorption of food.

Pancreatic Insufficiency

See page 85.

Tumours

In general, intestinal tumours tend to produce vomiting rather than diarrhoea. However, lymphosarcoma causes a diffuse thickening and destruction of the intestine by the deposition of white blood cells in the intestinal wall, and it can cause vomiting and/or diarrhoea. Lymphosarcoma can only be diagnosed by an intestinal biopsy. Chemotherapy may provide relief but not a cure, and as the tumour is malignant, surgery is usually unsuccessful.

Parasitic Worms

A heavy worm burden will produce diarrhoea, particularly in puppies. Parasitic worms are discussed in greater detail later in this chapter (*see* pages 87–90).

Vomiting and Diarrhoea

Gastroenteritis

Many infections and toxic substances produce inflammation of both the stomach and intestine. The onset is often sudden, with the patient vomiting and becoming depressed. His vomit may contain undigested food, even blood, and as the inflammation passes along the bowel, the dog develops diarrhoea.

The severity of symptoms can vary greatly. Mild cases may clear up spontaneously in a few hours but the more severe forms caused by parvovirus, for example, can produce severe dehydration and death within a few days.

Treatment Whether the gastroenteritis is severe or mild, all food must be withheld for twenty-four hours but it is essential to provide water. In severe or persistent cases, antibiotics and drugs to prevent vomiting and slow down bowel movements may be needed. Great care must be taken to avoid

dehydration and, in mild cases, fluids by mouth may be sufficient. If the dog refuses to drink, it will be necessary to hospitalise him and drip feed fluids into a vein, until he starts to drink again without vomiting.

Haemorrhagic Gastroenteritis

This tends to be a disease of the smaller breeds. Often, there is no obvious cause although an acute allergy is a possibility. The onset of blood-tinged vomiting and diarrhoea is very rapid and this diarrhoea can very quickly change to pure blood with the result that the dog becomes shocked. There is no rise in temperature but the dog will be depressed and off his food.

Treatment Any small dog with a haemorrhagic gastroenteritis needs immediate treatment. Solid food should be withheld and antibiotics and possibly anti-inflammatory drugs may be injected by the vet. If the dog is becoming shocked, hospitalisation and blood replacement fluids will be necessary.

Straining and Constipation

Straining occurs when the dog has to use greater than normal effort to evacuate his bowels or bladder. You must watch your dog carefully to see whether he is trying to pass faeces or urine. Constipation occurs when there is an accumulation of faeces in the rectum.

Constipation is very uncommon in the dog without any underlying disease which narrows the rectum. Such diseases include fractures of the pelvis, an enlarged prostate gland and tumours of the rectal wall. The most common cause of constipation is seen in the old, male dog with an enlarged prostate gland who has been chewing bones. The bone fragments then become obstructed at the level of the prostate. If the blockage is not removed, faeces build up in front of this and the dog will start to vomit.

Treatment The dog is usually anaesthetised and the impacted faeces are removed by the vet using an enema. Once the faeces are removed, the underlying cause must be treated. If the cause was a fractured pelvis, the future diet must be low in fibre, with no bones. Prostatic disease is discussed more fully in Chapter 15 (*see* page 184). Tumours are usually inoperable in this area.

Occasionally, in the old male dog the muscle supporting the rectum under the tail breaks down, allowing the rectum to bulge on either side of the anus below the tail. This is called a perineal hernia. Faeces accumulate in the hernia causing the dog to strain. Surgical repair of the hernia is usually successful although due to the fragility of the muscle tissue, the repair will sometimes break down.

Straining can also occur because of irritation to the lining of the rectum. This occurs through severe, persistent diarrhoea or small rectal tumours. Straining will cease once the diarrhoea has been controlled. Small tumours can often be removed surgically, or by cryosurgery, but larger ones are frequently inoperable.

PERITONITIS

Peritonitis is an inflammation of the lining membrane of the abdomen. It is an uncommon but serious disease. Peritonitis is characterised by a depressed dog who is off his food, with vomiting and diarrhoea, a raised temperature and severe abdominal pain. The infection can gain entry to the abdomen through a rupture of the intestinal wall, by a penetrating foreign body, from leakage of pus from an infected uterus, gunshot wounds or even, occasionally, from abdominal surgery.

Diagnosis of peritonitis is not always straightforward. The symptoms are often sufficient for a diagnosis, but sometimes it is necessary for the vet to perform an exploratory operation for a detailed examination.

Treatment Antibiotics are always required in the treatment of peritonitis but surgery may be required to repair any damage to the intestine, or remove an infected uterus. Excess pus can be flushed out with sterile saline. Severe peritonitis may leave the dog with scar tissue formation between the various organs in the abdomen. These adhesions may cause future complications such as narrowing of the intestine and this will make any future surgery difficult.

DISEASES OF THE PANCREAS

Acute Pancreatitis

This is a severe inflammation of the pancreas and produces similar symptoms to peritonitis. It is an extremely painful disease. Acute pancreatitis is diagnosed from the symptoms and blood tests.

Treatment Pancreatitis is treated with anti-inflammatory drugs and/or antibiotics. Food is withheld for a short period and then replaced with an easily digestible diet once the symptoms subside. Dogs which become dehydrated and shocked will require intravenous fluids in addition to other treatment.

Pancreatic Insufficiency

There are three causes of loss of pancreatic function:

1 The dog is born with a defective pancreas.
2 Repeated bouts of acute pancreatitis which slowly destroy the pancreas.
3 A slow degeneration of the pancreas. The

cause of this degeneration is unknown, but it is commonly seen in the German Shepherd Dog.

A dog with pancreatic insufficiency is unable to digest his food fully and this results in persistent diarrhoea, weight loss and a ravenous appetite.

Pancreatic insufficiency is diagnosed by laboratory testing of blood and faeces.

Treatment Pancreatic insufficiency is treated with replacement pancreatic enzymes mixed in the food and a change to an easily digestible diet. Prescription diets for this condition are available from your vet.

Tumours

The pancreas is a common site for tumour formation and these will often become quite large before they cause problems. As the pancreatic and bile ducts enter the intestine close together, tumours of the pancreas can cause an obstruction of the bile duct which leads to liver failure. The symptoms these tumours produce will, therefore, often be similar to those of liver failure.

Treatment Pancreatic tumours are very malignant and are usually inoperable, so euthanasia is normally recommended.

Diabetes Mellitus

Diabetes mellitus occurs when the blood sugar level rises above a certain level, causing an overspill of sugar into the urine through the kidneys. The glucose level in a normal dog is controlled by the hormone, insulin, which is produced in special small areas of tissue in the pancreas, the islets of Langerhans. If these areas fail to produce sufficient insulin, the dog develops clinical signs of diabetes.

Diabetes is much more common in overweight, entire bitches than in thin or spayed bitches or in dogs. A patient may start to lose weight but her appetite will increase, and because she loses water with the glucose in the urine, she becomes thirsty. Thus, a typical dog with diabetes is lethargic and has a markedly increased appetite and water intake.

Diabetes mellitus is diagnosed by testing the urine or blood for sugar levels.

Treatment If diabetes is diagnosed in entire bitches, the bitch should be spayed. This may completely correct the diabetes or, at least, make treatment easier because bitches tend to become destabilised during a heat period. Dietary management of diabetes is not as successful in the dog as in man, and most diabetic dogs require daily insulin injections. The injections must, of course, be given by the owner and are completely painless and simple to administer. The vet will often stabilise the bitch on the correct dose of insulin while demonstrating injection techniques to the owner, ensuring the owner can give the injection competently. It must be realised that a certain amount of time must be spent each day in testing urine, injecting insulin and sterilising syringes. A regular amount of food must be fed at the same time each day, usually immediately after the insulin injection. Once the blood glucose is stabilised, many dogs live quite happily for a normal life span as long as they have their daily injections of insulin.

If too much insulin is administered in error, the dog may go into a coma. The answer is to give glucose by mouth immediately. If diabetes is left untreated, or not enough daily insulin is given, toxic substances build up in the bloodstream and these will cause collapse and death of the dog. Even with treatment, many dogs with diabetes develop cataracts in their eyes.

DISEASES OF THE LIVER

Infection (Hepatitis)

The two most common causes of liver infection are infectious canine hepatitis and leptospirosis. These two diseases are discussed in Chapter 5 (*see* pages 63 and 65 respectively). As they are included in routine vaccination, neither infectious hepatitis nor leptospirosis are commonly seen.

Chronic Liver Failure

This is a common problem in the older dog and causes include cirrhosis, heart failure and tumours. Chronic liver failure can manifest itself in several ways but the most common feature is weight loss. There may be an increase in abdominal size, due to an increase in the size of the liver, or because of fluid accumulation (dropsy or ascites). As the disease progresses, the dog will have a poor appetite, an increased thirst, and he will possibly vomit and have diarrhoea. Occasionally jaundice will be seen.

Liver disease is not always easy to diagnose. It may be possible for the vet to feel the enlarged liver through the body wall and X-rays may demonstrate a change in liver size. However, a definite diagnosis may depend on blood tests or even a liver biopsy.

Treatment   Chronic liver disease is generally not curable, but the administration of specific vitamins, anabolic steroids and special fat-free diets may often reduce the symptoms and prolong the dog's active life. Prescription diets for this condition are available from the vet.

Tumours

Liver tumours are common, either as primary tumours, or secondaries which have spread from malignant tumours in other parts of the body. The symptoms are those of chronic liver failure.

X-rays will usually reveal the tumour although an exploratory operation to inspect the liver may be necessary.

Treatment   If the tumour is confined to one part of the liver, it may be possible to remove it surgically. In the vast majority of cases, however, the tumour is widespread throughout the liver and euthanasia is necessary.

PARASITIC INTESTINAL WORMS

There are two types of parasitic worms which infect the intestines of dogs – roundworms and tapeworms – and these include three species of roundworm and three species of tapeworm.

Roundworms

Toxocara Canis

This is the common ascarid roundworm which is readily seen in either the faeces or, occasionally, in the vomit of puppies. They are round, white, often coiled and up to 20cm (8in) long. These are the adult worms which live in the small intestine of puppies and to a lesser degree in mature dogs. Once they are voided in the faeces they die, but while in the intestine they breed by laying microscopic eggs. These are passed, unnoticed by the owner, in the faeces in their thousands, and due to a very tough outer shell can survive in the environment for well over a year, long after the faeces have been washed away. After about three weeks, the egg develops to an infectious larval stage, still within the shell, and if this is taken in by a puppy and swallowed, the larva burrows through the

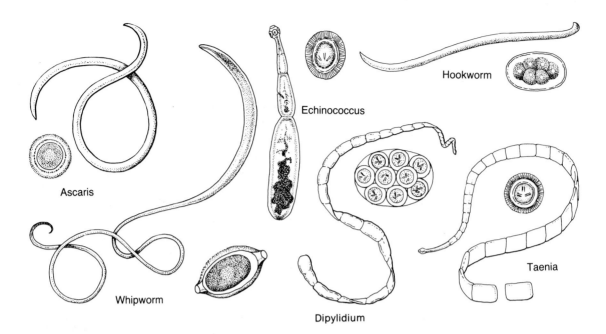

Fig 11 Parasitic worms and their eggs (not to scale)

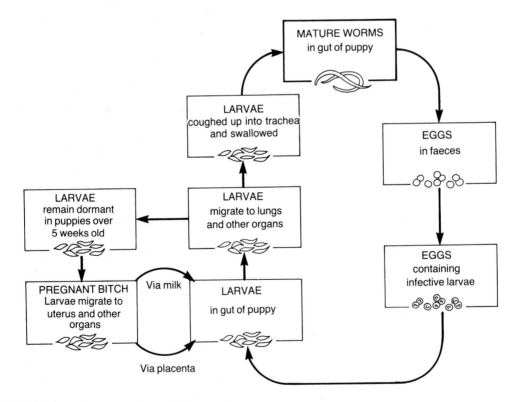

Fig 12 Life cycle of the dog roundworm (Toxocara canis)

intestine wall and enters the bloodstream. Most larvae are then carried to the lungs which they may damage, causing a cough. In young puppies under twelve weeks of age the larvae are coughed up and swallowed. They then develop in the bowel into adult *Toxocara* roundworms and begin to breed and lay eggs to complete the life cycle.

Dogs over the age of roughly three months develop an age immunity to the larvae which, after burrowing through the intestine wall and entering the blood stream, are not coughed up and swallowed, but transported by the bloodstream all over the body. When a capillary (small end blood vessel) is reached, they burrow out and form a minute cyst in the organ in which they find themselves. This is frequently a muscle. These small cysts cause no symptoms at all and in a dog remain dormant and unchanged for the rest of their lives. In a female, these cysts remain dormant until the bitch is pregnant, when the hormone levels stimulate the larvae to become active again. They burrow out of their cysts, into the bloodstream and are transported into the wall of the uterus and across the placenta into the developing foetus. This complicated life cycle ensures that almost all puppies are born already infected with *Toxocara* roundworms.

In addition, the larvae migrate to the mammary glands and infect the young puppies when they suckle the bitch.

Thus the main sources of roundworm infestation are the pregnant and lactating bitch, and young puppies that are passing infected faeces. These faeces, however, are not infective until they have been in the environment for three weeks.

Diagnosis   Where worming has not been carried out, or the effects of worming are to be assessed, the examination of faecal samples is useful. The vet will dilute a fresh faeces sample to separate any worm eggs, and then examine the sample under a microscope to confirm their presence or absence.

Treatment and prevention   Fresh faeces are not infectious and therefore should be picked up and disposed of before the eggs develop to the infective larval stage.

The bitch should be wormed before mating, at or after forty-five days pregnant, a day or so after whelping and every two weeks after that until the puppies are twelve weeks old, with a larvicidal wormer from your vet so that any larvae migrating through her body tissues will also be killed.

The puppies should be wormed at two weeks of age and thereafter every two weeks until they are twelve weeks old using a safe but effective worm medicine. Preferably this should be a syrup to start with, but a tablet or granule form can be used once they are weaned. Worming should continue at four, five and six months of age. After this age **all** dogs should be wormed every three to six months of their life.

Human infection   Very, very occasionally the *Toxocara* worm will affect a child who contacts the infective larvae on the ground, three weeks after they were passed by a dog, and then licks his fingers. In the vast majority of cases any larvae swallowed are killed by the stomach acids but very rarely one survives to be carried by the bloodstream to an organ such as the eye where it lodges in the optic nerve. This can cause loss of vision in the affected eye which may be partial or total. To prevent this unlikely occurrence, dogs should be wormed thoroughly and regularly, and faeces picked up and disposed of.

It is impossible for dog roundworms to infect children's bowels so any worms seen here are human parasitic worms passed from person to person. It should also be noted that it is impossible for children or dogs to become infected with *Toxocara* either from fresh faeces or from handling or being licked by a dog. The egg must develop for three weeks before it is infectious.

Hookworms

These worms are far less common than *Toxocara* and mainly occur in kennels with a hygiene problem. They are much shorter, thinner, greyish red and up to about 3cm (1in) long. The eggs hatch in moist ground into larvae which gain entry to a dog by penetrating the feet or the skin where they may cause a local irritation, or by ingestion. Large numbers will cause diarrhoea and anaemia. Their presence can be diagnosed by faeces examination, and the worms can be killed with modern worming medicine.

Whipworms

These worms are also uncommon and live in the large intestine. Whipworms are about 5cm (2in) long with a narrow front end and thicker rear part, hence the name. Infection is by the ingestion of the larvae and, like hookworms, occurs more commonly in dogs in dirty kennels. Whipworms can cause diarrhoea but this is rarely severe. Infestation is diagnosed by examination of the faeces and the adult worms can be killed with modern worming medicine.

Tapeworms

Dipylidium

This tapeworm is fairly common in the dog. It can grow up to 50cm (20in) long and consists of a small pointed head and a long flattened segmented body. The head of the tapeworm becomes embedded in the intestinal wall and, as the tapeworm grows from its head or scolex, it produces segments. These break off at the rear of the worm to appear around the dog's anus or on his faeces. Initially, these move like a caterpillar but soon dry to look like rice grains. These segments are full of eggs which are released into the environment. Development into cysts continues once the eggs are ingested by a dog flea, the intermediate host. The dog then becomes infected by eating the flea. There is no direct spread from dog to dog.

Taenia

This tapeworm is 1–2m (3–6ft) long, a much longer tapeworm than *Dipylidium*. The intermediate hosts include mice, hares, rabbits and sheep which the dog must eat raw to become infected.

Echinococcus

This is not a very common tapeworm and is usually confined to certain areas of the country. It is very small, less than 1cm (½in) in length and has only three or four segments. The intermediate hosts include man, domestic farm animals and wild animals, and in these hosts the tapeworm forms large harmful cysts, called hydatid cysts.

Adult tapeworms are comparatively harmless to the dog but large numbers will occasionally produce diarrhoea and weight loss. *Echinococcus* cysts can be a serious problem in man.

Diagnosis Except in the case of *Echinococcus*, the tapeworm segments may be seen around the anus and if infection is in doubt, eggs can be detected in the faeces by the vet using a microscope.

Treatment Adult tapeworms are not easily killed although modern drugs are proving successful. Infection can be prevented by regular treatment for fleas, cooking of suspect meat and keeping dogs away from all carrion. Dogs such as terriers, who catch and eat small rodents, should be treated on a regular basis.

7 The Respiratory System

The respiratory system is composed of the nose, the larynx, the pharynx, the trachea, the bronchi and the lungs. It has two functions, firstly gaseous exchange, to provide the body with oxygen and at the same time to remove carbon dioxide; and secondly temperature regulation by panting as the dog is unable to lose heat by sweating.

NORMAL STRUCTURE AND FUNCTION

The nose is a bony box containing a myriad of fine bones covered with a blood-rich membrane. Air is drawn into the nose through the nostrils, where it is warmed and filtered of dust and foreign particles. This warmed, clean air then passes across the pharynx into the larynx. During swallowing, the entrance to the larynx is protected by a flap of cartilage, called the epiglottis, which prevents food particles from being inhaled. The larynx contains the vocal cords which, in addition to producing sound, can be closed to prevent food and water from entering the lungs. The larynx leads down into the trachea, which is simply a non-collapsible tube running the length of the neck. The trachea divides at the level of the heart into two bronchi, one of which enters each lung. These bronchi subdivide into smaller bronchi, then bronchioles, which terminate into thin-walled air sacs, or alveoli. The walls of the alveoli are richly supplied with blood vessels and it is here that the exchange of oxygen and carbon dioxide occurs.

The lower trachea, bronchi and lungs are contained within the chest walls and dia-phragm (a thin sheet of muscle between the chest and abdomen). During inspiration the chest expands as the ribs move outwards and the diaphragm moves downwards. During expiration, the chest contracts as the chest wall relaxes to its resting position.

A dog's resting respiratory rate varies from ten to thirty breaths per minute, depending on the breed and age. In the normal resting dog, breathing will be

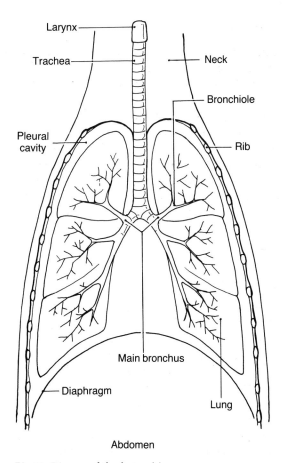

Fig 13 Diagram of the chest and lungs

Labels: Larynx, Trachea, Neck, Bronchiole, Pleural cavity, Rib, Main bronchus, Diaphragm, Lung, Abdomen

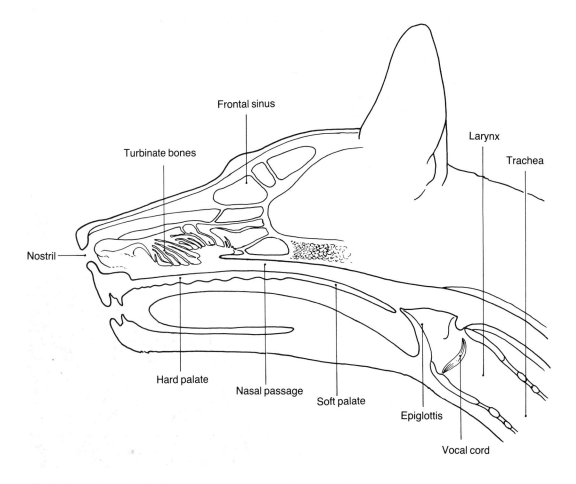

Fig 14 *Section through the head to show the main structures of the nose and larynx*

shallow and regular and the tongue and gums will be pink. A dog with severe oxygen shortage will have exaggerated, rapid breathing even at rest, and the tongue and gums will be a blue colour. Such a dog is said to be cyanotic. It must be remembered that the gums and mouth of Chows are always blue, due to pigment. In this breed the blue coloration is normal.

DISEASES OF THE NOSE

Infection (Rhinitis)

Nasal infections are fairly common in the dog. They can be caused by viruses, bacteria and fungi. Some nasal infections may be part of a more widespread disease such as distemper or kennel cough.

The first sign that a dog has an infected nose is usually sneezing, often accompanied by a watery discharge. As the disease progresses, the sneezing becomes more frequent and the discharge may become purulent or bloodstained. This may adhere

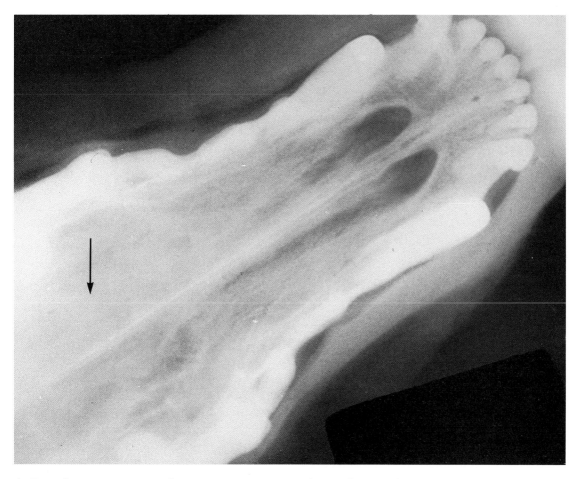

An X-ray of a tumour in the nose of a mongrel. The air spaces are obliterated on one side of the muzzle.

around the nostril and the resulting nasal obstruction often leads to mouth breathing. The signs of nasal infection are usually self-evident, although the cause may be difficult to diagnose.

Treatment   Rhinitis is often treated with antibiotics but, if there is no response, X-rays and laboratory testing may be necessary to identify the cause. Fungal infection and well established bacterial infections are difficult to treat and they may require surgical drainage of the nose.

Foreign Bodies

Due to the dog's habitual sniffing, grass seeds and other foreign objects may be inhaled through the nostrils. The dog will start to sneeze violently, usually after a walk through long grass, and in the early stages the tip of the seed may be seen protruding from the nostril. It should be carefully removed with a pair of tweezers. If the seed is not removed, and migrates further into the nose, a bloodstained purulent discharge will appear at the affected nostril within a day or so. It is essential that the dog is taken

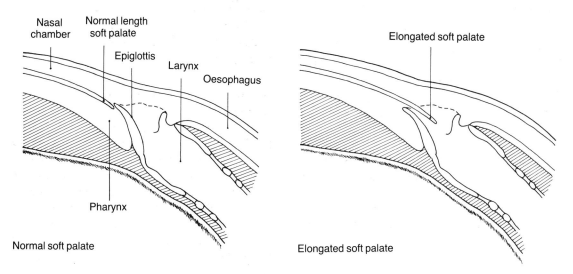

Fig 15 *An elongated soft palate obstructs the entrance to the larynx*

to a vet as the foreign body must be removed as soon as possible under anaesthetic.

Tumours

These are fairly common in the larger breeds such as the Old English Sheepdog. The first sign is usually an intermittent haemorrhage from one nostril, and X-rays may reveal a mass in one or both nasal chambers. Most tumours of the nose are highly malignant and surgery is difficult and of little value.

DISEASES PRODUCING NOISY RESPIRATION

Noisy breathing is the result of a partial obstruction of the airway anywhere between the nostrils and the lungs. It is a major problem in the short-nosed breeds, such as the Pekingese and Pug. The shorter the nose the worse the problem, because although all the normal structures are present in these breeds, they are forced to occupy a much shorter space, thus producing overcrowding and narrowing of the airway. Often the

cause is not just a single factor but one problem leading to another.

Narrow Nostrils (Stenosis)

This is a common problem in the Bulldog and Pekingese. During inspiration, the nostril can almost become occluded, and surgery may be required.

Elongated Soft Palate

This is a common condition in which the relatively over-long soft palate partially obstructs the entrance to the larynx. The dog makes an intermittent snorting noise and may cough frequently in an attempt to clear the larynx.

Treatment In most cases, surgery to shorten the soft palate is helpful and eliminates the obstruction. We have seen it most often in the Cavalier King Charles Spaniel.

Collapse of the Trachea and Larynx

This collapse can occur as a result of a higher obstruction, such as an elongated soft palate, and is seen more often in the very small breeds. Affected dogs will have a very harsh, laboured inspiration and a cough.

Treatment   Surgery is the only treatment likely to be successful. Small, sterile, plastic rings are placed at intervals along the collapsed portion of the trachea. An open airway is maintained by suturing the trachea to these rings.

Laryngeal Paralysis

Unlike the previous condition, this is a disease of the old dog, and we have seen it most frequently in the Labrador. A snoring noise is heard on inspiration and is caused by the air vibrating the loose and paralysed vocal cords which are obstructing the airway. Under certain circumstances, such as hot weather, laryngeal paralysis can produce an almost complete blockage of the larynx. An affected dog will gasp for air with his mouth wide open and may even become cyanotic and collapse.

Treatment   If the paralysis is severe, symptoms can be eliminated by a surgical operation to prevent the vocal cords from occluding the airway.

DISEASES PRODUCING A COUGH

The cough is a reflex which, by forcing air quickly out of the chest, clears irritating foreign matter from the bronchi, trachea and larynx. Severe inflammation of these structures will also stimulate the cough reflex.

Acute Inflammation of the Larynx, Trachea and Bronchi (Laryngitis, Tracheitis and Bronchitis)

Inflammation of these structures can be caused by an infection such as kennel cough or canine distemper, by irritant fumes or by foreign material. Usually, all three parts of the airway are affected at the same time.

The onset of coughing can be so sudden that the owner thinks that the dog has a bone lodged in his throat. In most cases, the patient is still relatively well and in the early stages he will continue to eat. If the larynx is affected there may be a temporary loss of voice.

Treatment   These acute infections respond readily to cough medicines or antibiotics. Rest is essential and exercise should be severely restricted until the dog has recovered. Some respiratory conditions are highly infectious and affected dogs should be isolated until the cough has disappeared.

Chronic Bronchitis

Chronic bronchitis is a major problem in the older dog. It is caused by a persistent, low grade infection, or irritation, which produces irreversible changes in the bronchi. In the majority of cases the cough develops slowly and, at first, may be present only on exertion. Many cases will not develop further but in a few, the frequency increases until the dog seems to cough almost constantly. Chronic bronchitis then becomes a very debilitating disease.

Treatment   There is no cure, but a combination of antibiotics, anti-inflammatory drugs, bronchodilators and drugs to break up the mucus can greatly reduce the amount of coughing and improve the quality of life.

95

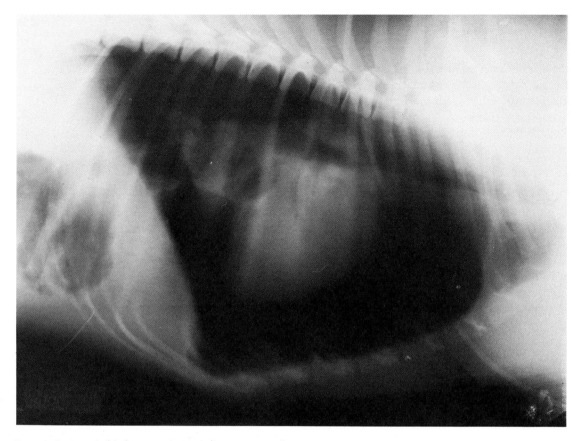

Pneumothorax – the black area on the X-ray shows air around the lungs.

Lung Worms

These worms cause the formation of small nodules in the trachea, usually where it divides into the bronchi, which cause an intermittent cough. Occasionally, the nodules can become so large that they obstruct the airway. The condition is diagnosed by the vet examining the trachea with an endoscope under a general anaesthetic, or by X-rays which reveal the nodules.

Treatment Modern parasitic drugs are required from your vet to kill the worms.

Foreign Bodies

These are extremely uncommon but when seen can include bits of twig, grass seeds or the inhalation of vomit. Foreign bodies produce a harsh, dry cough which begins suddenly. Some foreign bodies can be difficult to locate in a dog who is under a general anaesthetic even after a thorough examination of the trachea and bronchi using an endoscope.

Treatment The foreign body must be removed with long forceps to prevent its presence leading to suffocation or pneumonia.

DISEASES PRODUCING LABOURED BREATHING

Diseases which produce laboured breathing are normally those diseases which occupy space within the chest, thus reducing the volume of lung tissue available for oxygenation of the blood.

Pneumonia

This is an infection of the lung tissue which produces an inflammatory reaction in the air sacs. Pneumonia is uncommon in the dog but can be caused by viruses, bacteria, fungi or foreign material. It is seen more commonly as part of a generalised disease such as canine distemper.

A dog with pneumonia will be quiet and off his food, he will have a raised temperature and a marked respiratory effort. If the inflammation affects the bronchi, there will also be a cough. A diagnosis is usually made by the vet who takes into account clinical signs, examines the chest with a stethoscope and may confirm the diagnosis with an X-ray of the chest.

Treatment High dosages of antibiotics are required in the treatment of pneumonia, and in severe cases oxygen therapy may also be needed. Rest is essential.

Accidents

Respiratory failure is a common sequel to trauma, especially road traffic accidents. There are several types of injury that may be encountered and they all result in a dog who is depressed and has laboured breathing. The various injuries are diagnosed by clinical and X-ray examination. After an accident, chest injuries must be corrected first, as a priority to maintain life, before treatment for other injuries, such as fractured legs, are dealt with.

Haemorrhage into the Lung

Rupture of a blood vessel in the lung will release blood which fills the air sacs. The dog will have laboured breathing, may cough up blood and will have pale mucous membranes. A severe haemorrhage may result in death as the lungs can rapidly fill with blood.

Treatment Treatment is difficult as this free blood cannot easily be removed. The dog must remain quiet and still until his own defence mechanisms remove the blood clot. If he survives, he should show a marked improvement after a few days as the blood is absorbed and breathing becomes easier.

Rupture of a Lung

Sometimes a broken rib will penetrate a lung, or a lung may be ruptured by the force of the accident. In either case, free air will be released into the chest cavity and this will occupy space which would normally be occupied by the lungs. The chest will sound hollow when tapped with a finger. A diagnosis is made by an X-ray examination which will show air around the lungs, and possibly a broken rib. This condition is called pneumothorax.

Treatment This air can be drained from the chest cavity by the insertion of a drainage tube. In most cases, the tear in the lung will heal without surgery, unless a fractured rib is depressed inwards and aggravates the condition.

Ruptured Diaphragm

Rupture of the diaphragm will allow abdominal contents, such as the liver, spleen or intestine, to move forward into the chest cavity. The chest will sound dull when the vet listens to it with a stethoscope and the

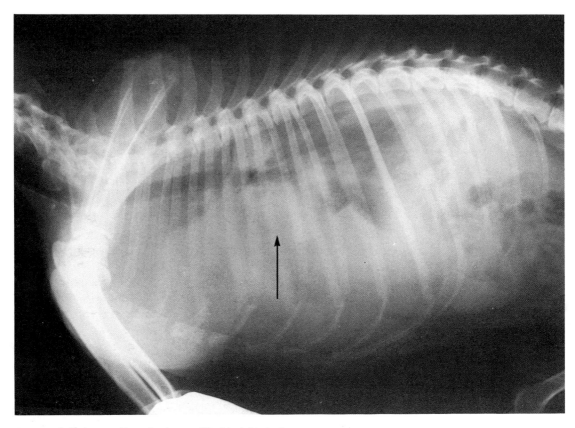

A ruptured diaphragm allows the chest to fill with abdominal organs.

abdominal contents will be seen in the chest on an X-ray.

Treatment Surgery is required both to replace these organs in their normal position and to repair the tear in the diaphragm. Close circuit anaesthesia with positive pressure is essential as, due to the rupture of the diaphragm, once the abdominal incision is made, the chest cavity is connected to the outside air, and the dog is, therefore, unable to breathe for himself.

Tumours

Chest tumours can cause respiratory embarrassment both by occupying lung space and by causing the accumulation of fluid within the chest. Primary tumours arising from the lung tissue are uncommon but the lungs are a common site for tumour spread from other parts of the body.

Treatment Lung tumours are nearly always malignant and inoperable, and euthanasia is essential once the dog becomes distressed. Occasionally chemotherapy can help.

8 The Circulatory System

The circulatory system can be regarded as a continuous tube running in a figure of eight with the heart at the cross-over point. One loop supplies the lungs while the other supplies all the other tissues of the body. The circulating blood provides the body with a transportation system.

NORMAL STRUCTURE AND FUNCTION

The heart is a muscular, four-chambered pump and its sole function is the propulsion of blood around the body. Thick-walled, elastic blood vessels, the arteries, carry blood away from the heart, and the veins, which have thin walls, return blood from the tissues to the heart. The blood pressure is much higher in the arteries than in the veins.

The strength and rate of the heartbeat is controlled by a very small area of heart tissue, called the sinoatrial node, situated in the wall of the right atrium. This area releases electrical impulses which spread through the heart and cause it to contract in such a way that blood is forced out through the arteries. This spread of electrical activity can be measured and the recording is known as an electrocardiograph (ECG). The sinoatrial node receives nerve messages from the brain through the autonomic nervous system and these messages will change the rate and strength of the heart beat. After all, a dog requires a greater cardiac output when he is running than at rest.

Unoxygenated blood (blood low in oxygen) leaves the right ventricle of the heart through the pulmonary artery to the lungs.

Here the blood exchanges its carbon dioxide for oxygen and returns to the left atrium of the heart through the pulmonary vein. This blood is pumped into the left ventricle and from here through the aorta to all the other organs of the body, such as the brain, muscles and liver. In these organs, oxygen and nutrients are extracted from the blood and new nutrients enter the bloodstream from the breakdown of food in the intestine. The blood returns via a large vein, the vena cava, to the right atrium and from here to the right ventricle, and then the lungs to begin the cycle again. The carotid artery, one of the first branches of the aorta, is the main arterial supply to the brain, and the jugular vein returns the blood to the heart after it has circulated through the brain.

Blood is composed of a fluid, the plasma, which has suspended in it blood cells. Red blood cells contain a substance, haemoglobin, which combines with oxygen to transport it round the body. White blood cells attack and rid the body of infections and other foreign material. Platelets and other clotting substances in the blood are required for the control of haemorrhage. Food and hormones are carried in the plasma. Most red and white blood cells are produced in the red bone marrow. A few white blood cells are, however, produced in the lymph nodes, thymus and spleen.

A second circulating system, the lymphatic system, is responsible for combating infection and also for returning fluid to the heart which has leaked from the blood vessels. Lymph nodes are composed of white blood cells and they are scattered throughout the body. The superficial lymph nodes can be felt underneath the skin, for example under

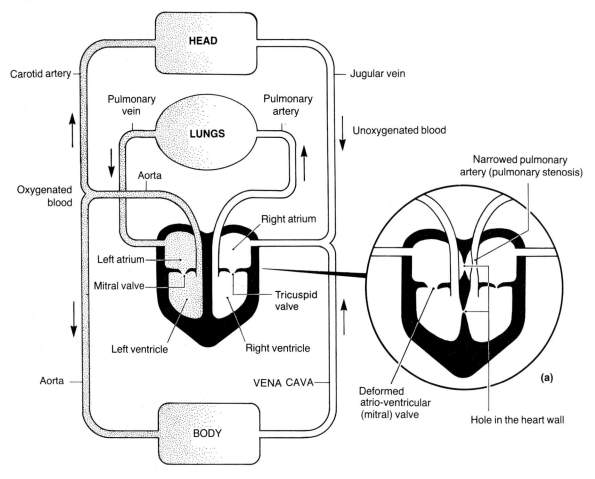

*Fig 16 Schematic diagram of the circulatory system
(a) common congenital heart defects*

CONGENITAL HEART DISEASE

See Chapter 4, The Growing Dog, page 53.

ACQUIRED HEART DISEASE

Acquired heart failure is not a major problem in the dog. It tends to occur in the old dog although in the Cavalier King Charles Spaniel and giant breeds it can occur in middle age. Dogs have a large cardiac reserve and heart disease is often well advanced before signs of heart failure appear.

the throat. The tonsils are similar in structure and function to the lymph nodes. The vet will often feel these nodes for evidence of enlargement which may indicate disease. The spleen, a large organ situated alongside the stomach in the abdomen, is part of the lymphatic system and helps fight disease as well as acting as a store for red blood cells. The thymus is composed of white blood cells and is situated in the entrance to the chest. It is fairly large in the young dog and helps fight disease but in the adult it almost disappears.

Causes

Valve Damage

In the dog this is the most common cause of heart failure. In the old dog heart valves slowly thicken with time and become less efficient until they can no longer function correctly. The mitral or left valve is the one most commonly affected.

Endocarditis (inflammation of the heart valves), can also lead to valvular incompetence. This is usually caused by a blood borne infection.

Diseases of the Heart Muscle

These are fairly rare but include tumours, infection, injury and, in the giant breeds, an inefficient enlargement of the heart muscle of unknown cause.

Disorders of Conduction

Sometimes there is a localised damage to the heart muscle affecting a specific area which is responsible for the normal rhythm and heart rate. Damage to this area can result in a heart which beats too fast, too slow or very unevenly.

Signs of Heart Failure

Heart failure occurs when the heart is unable to maintain an adequate blood supply to the tissues of the body. Heart attacks, as seen in man, do not occur in the dog and most heart disease tends to be degenerative and progressive. In the early stages of heart damage, the heart is able to maintain output by increasing in size and by an increase in heart rate.

The signs of heart disease vary depending

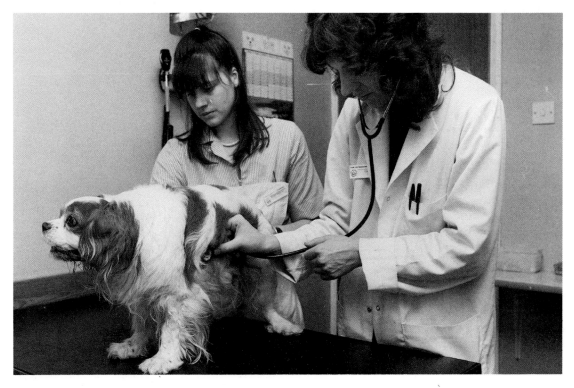

A stethoscope in use on a Cavalier King Charles Spaniel with valvular heart disease.

on whether the left or right side of the heart is failing.

Left-Sided Heart Failure

Left-sided heart failure is more common and produces mainly respiratory signs. The first sign is an occasional cough on exercise but, as heart failure progresses and more fluid accumulates in the lungs, this cough worsens until it is persistent. The dog will lose weight and be less able to exercise. In the final stages he will have severe respiratory embarrassment, may be coughing up a pink, frothy fluid and will be severely cyanosed.

Right-Sided Heart Failure

Right-sided heart failure produces congestion of the abdominal organs which results in poor digestion, poor kidney function, an enlarged liver and ascites (the accumulation of fluid in the abdomen). There is also severe weight loss and the dog tires easily on exercise.

Sudden collapse from heart disease is uncommon. It can occur in heart conditions where there is an irregular beat. On occasions, the heart rate drops so low that the heart almost stops. Fainting attacks are sometimes seen in Boxers, due to excessive activity in the nerve which slows heart rate.

Diagnosis By listening to the heart through a stethoscope, the vet will be able to hear if the heart has any defects, such as heart murmurs, heart enlargement and an irregular or fast heartbeat. He will also feel the pulse with finger pressure on the inside of the thigh to see if this is weak – an

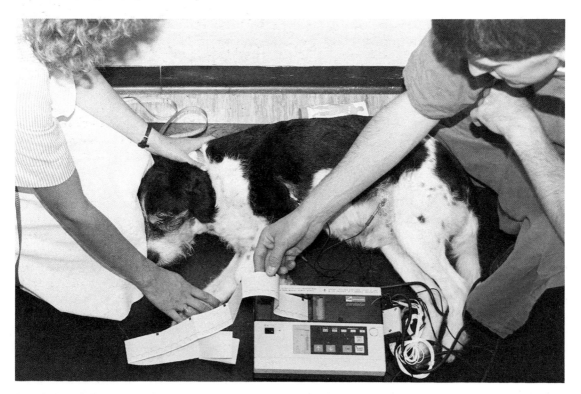

An ECG recording in progress.

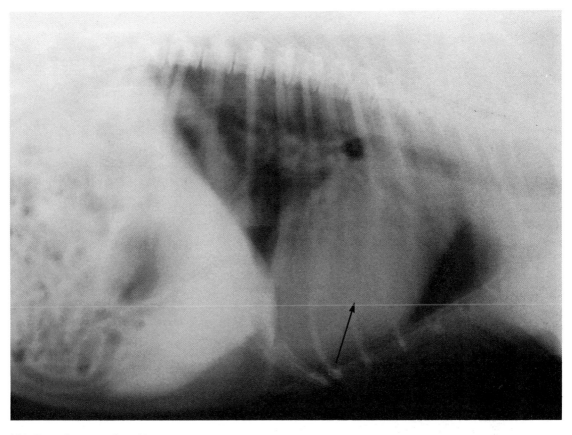

This X-ray shows an enlarged heart.

indication of poor cardiac output. In many cases, the examination of the heart sounds, along with the other clinical signs, may be enough to make a diagnosis of heart failure. In more complicated cases it will be necessary for the vet to X-ray the dog's chest to detect any abnormality in the size or shape of the heart. An ECG machine is also a useful aid in the diagnosis of heart conditions.

Ultrasound scanning is gradually becoming available to the veterinary profession and is proving very useful in diagnosis of heart disorders, especially at specialist referral centres. The heart can be seen actually functioning on a video monitor and detail recorded of the valve function. We are certain this method of diagnosis will become

more widespread in heart conditions as it is easily performed on a conscious dog and has no harmful effects on either the patient or operator.

Treatment Once heart failure has been diagnosed the work load of the heart must be kept to a minimum, which means reducing exercise. In severe cases, it may be necessary to make the dog rest in a cage until the heart is stabilised. If the dog is overweight, this excess weight must be shed as a matter of urgency to reduce the load on the heart.

Excessive salt in the diet will contribute to fluid build up in the lungs or abdomen, so heart patients require a salt-free diet. This means either feeding a specially formu-

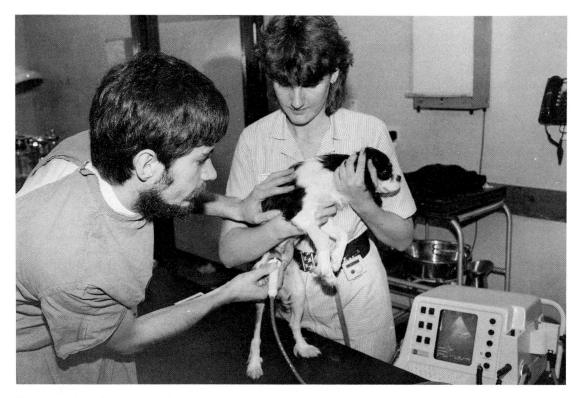

An ultrasound scan in progress.

lated prescription diet available from the vet or the owner must prepare his dog's own diet of fresh meat, vegetables and rice with no salt added.

Diuretics are very valuable in the treatment of heart diseases as they remove the accumulated excess fluid. They can be given either intermittently or continuously, depending on the degree of fluid accumulation. Care must be taken as excessive fluid loss will cause dehydration.

Some dogs will require treatment with digitalis derivatives to increase the strength of the heart beat, while at the same time reducing the heart rate. Dogs with irregular heart rates can be treated with drugs to stabilise this and, in special circumstances, pace-makers can be fitted.

Old dogs with heart failure cannot be treated routinely by surgery to correct the heart defect. However, by close monitoring of exercise, feeding the correct diet and using drugs carefully, their useful happy life can be extended.

HEARTWORM

This is a common cause of heart disease in warmer countries and is caused by small parasitic worms which live in the arteries of the lungs. The presence of these worms causes a blockage to the blood flow through the lungs which increases the pressure on the right side of the heart and leads to right-sided heart failure. The dog becomes infected with the heartworm larvae through the bite of an infected mosquito. Heartworm is diagnosed by the vet examining a drop of blood under the microscope for the heartworm larvae.

Heartworm infestation is difficult to treat. If congestive heart failure has developed, no attempt should be made to kill the heartworms but the dog should be treated for congestive heart failure.

In mildly affected dogs the adult heartworms are killed with a special drug, which has to be used very carefully as the dying worms can increase the damage to the lungs. Once the adult heartworms are killed, the larvae circulating in the bloodstream are killed using a different drug. Heartworm infection can be prevented by regular treatment to kill any larvae in the circulation before they develop into adult heartworms.

ANAEMIA

Anaemia is caused by a fall in the number of circulating red blood cells in the bloodstream. The dog will appear pale and, in extreme cases, the gums and tongue will be almost white. He will be weak, reluctant to exercise, have a poor appetite and a fast respiratory rate.

Anaemia is uncommon in the dog and has several causes. Certain infections, such as leptospirosis, will cause anaemia while chronic liver and kidney disease may give rise to a mild form. Haemorrhage, especially small repeated haemorrhages, will steadily cause the loss of red blood cells from the circulation. This can be seen in warfarin poisoning (rat poisoning) or, commonly, from small tumours in the spleen. Tumours of the bone marrow will prevent the formation of new red blood cells and lead to anaemia as the circulating red blood cells reach the end of their 120-day life.

Although the clinical signs provide evidence of severe anaemia, confirmation is provided in the laboratory by the examination of a blood smear.

Treatment Any dog suffering from severe anaemia will require a blood transfusion to replace the lost blood cells but then the underlying cause must be attended to.

Vitamin K injections will be given for warfarin poisoning, haemorrhaging tumours may be surgically removed and infections treated with antibiotics.

BLOOD CLOTTING DEFECTS

Failure of the blood clotting mechanism is rare in the dog. It will result in severe haemorrhage, even from small wounds, and small spontaneous haemorrhages will occur in various parts of the body, especially in the joints and in the chest.

Affected dogs will be intermittently lame or may have difficulty in breathing depending on the site of the haemorrhage. The faeces and urine may contain blood and, as the problem progresses, the dog will become anaemic.

Haemophilia, as seen in man, does occur in the dog but it is extremely rare. Chronic liver disease may decrease the efficiency of blood clotting as the liver manufactures certain of the blood clotting substances. Poisons such as warfarin directly affect the blood clotting mechanisms. A fall in circulating platelets which are important in blood clotting will lead to a failure of this mechanism.

Blood clotting disorders can be diagnosed only by laboratory testing of blood, although warfarin poisoning can be diagnosed on clinical signs if rat poison has been used locally. The antidote is vitamin K. Low platelet counts can often be reversed by corticosteroid therapy.

LYMPHOSARCOMA/ LEUKAEMIA

Lymphosarcoma is a tumour of the white cells of the blood and is fairly common in the middle-aged and old dog. The affected white blood cells infiltrate various organs of the body to produce lymphosarcoma tumours. Very rarely there is an increase in the circulating white blood cells to produce leukaemia. The symptoms are governed by which organ is affected but lymphosarcoma develops slowly. The first signs are lethargy, often a poor appetite and weight loss. If the nervous system is affected the dog will become uncoordinated and weak. Infiltration of the lungs, liver or kidney will result in failure of these organs. Intestinal lymphosarcoma produces vomiting and diarrhoea. Often, lymphosarcoma will affect the lymph nodes around the body and produce large superficial lumps, especially under the throat.

Lymphosarcoma is not easily diagnosed from an examination of the blood and will often require a biopsy of the affected organ.

Treatment Lymphosarcoma can be treated with chemotherapy using anti-neoplastic drugs which kill tumour cells, as in the treatment of leukaemia in man. However, this treatment does not usually kill the tumour but may slow the progress of the disease for several months.

DISEASES OF THE SPLEEN

The spleen is rarely affected by disease but is frequently a site for tumour formation. Such tumours are fairly common in the old dog, can be either single or multiple and can become so large that they fill most of the abdomen. The dog becomes thin except for a large round abdomen. He will have a poor appetite and become lethargic. Splenic tumours rupture easily and haemorrhage into the abdomen and if this occurs, the first sign is a collapsed dog. The abdomen can become very distended through the accumulation of free blood and death can occur very rapidly.

Splenic tumours can be diagnosed by the vet when he palpates the abdomen and they will show up on an X-ray.

Treatment The entire spleen, along with the tumour, must be removed surgically by an operation called a splenectomy. This is a serious operation but, if successful, has no detrimental effect on the dog's health. A blood or plasma transfusion is normally necessary. However, some splenic tumours may spread to other organs and, if this has occurred, removing the spleen will be of little long-term benefit to the dog.

9 Skin and Associated Structures

The skin is the tough, outer, protective covering of the body and it has several functions. It protects the rest of the tissues of the body from dangers such as trauma and infection. The skin and hair together maintain the internal temperature of the body by insulating it from excessive heat and cold. Via nerve endings, the skin relays messages about the environment and warns of painful stimuli. It provides a waterproof layer for the body and is also important in water conservation.

NORMAL STRUCTURE AND FUNCTION

The skin is divided into two layers: the outer tough epidermis and the underlying dermis.

The epidermis is composed of flat, dead cells which are being constantly produced from the bottom layer and continuously worn away from the surface. In certain areas, where there is excessive wear and tear, such as the pads, the epidermis has become much

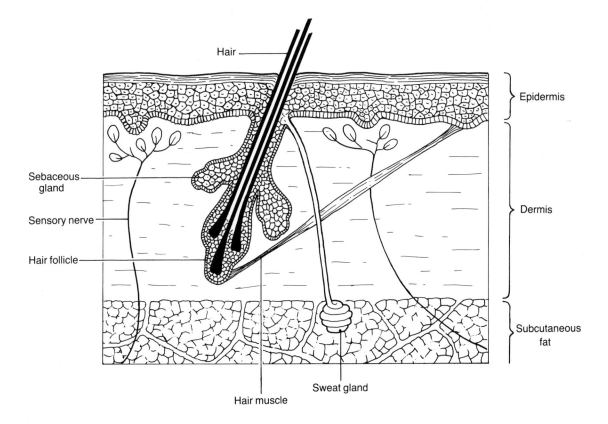

Hair

Epidermis

Sebaceous gland

Sensory nerve

Hair follicle

Dermis

Subcutaneous fat

Sweat gland

Hair muscle

Fig 17 Structure of the skin

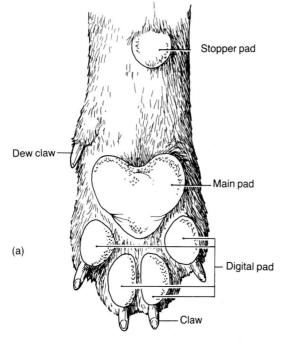

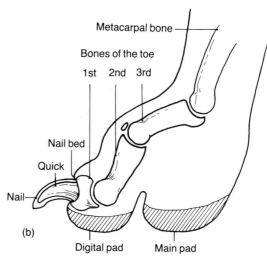

Fig 18 Structure of the foot
  (a) Arrangement of the pads in the forefoot
  (b) Section of the foot

thicker. This can also occur on the underside of the elbow and is seen more frequently in the heavier breeds where this skin becomes hairless and thickened.

The dermis is a thicker layer and contains the blood vessels, nerve endings, sweat glands and hair follicles. Each hair follicle has an associated small muscle, which when it contracts, produces erection of the hair.

Two areas of the skin have become very specialised:

1 The anal sacs are small scent glands which lie on either side and slightly below the anus. These sacs are normally emptied every time the dog defaecates and, in this way, the dog is able to mark his territory.
2 The nails are formed from a specialised part of the skin, the nail bed. The inner part of the nail, the quick, contains blood vessels and nerves.

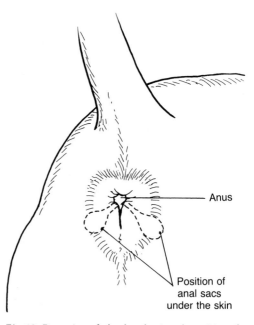

Fig 19 Rear view of the dog showing the position of the anal sacs

The skin, because of its protective role, is prone to disease so the vet in general practice will be called on to treat many skin problems. In fact, about thirty per cent of our case load in small animal practice concerns the skin.

As many skin diseases are a reaction between the dog's skin and his environment, many of these diseases become chronic, intermittent or seasonal and, as such, require constant or intermittent treatment. Many of these diseases cannot be cured because of the impracticality in changing the dog's environment, but they can be controlled.

DISEASES CAUSING ITCHING

Parasites

Fleas

Fleas are extremely common and are considered to be the single most common cause of skin disease. Adult fleas spend very little time on their host as they only jump on for long enough to have a feed of blood, perhaps four hours per day. They then jump off and spend the remainder of the day in carpets, cracks and crevices and even in the dog's bedding in the home, or in the grass and hedgerows outside the home. Given the right conditions, fleas can live for several months between feeds. The white eggs are not laid on the dog, but in the environment, and these hatch out into minute black maggot-like larvae. In the winter when the temperature is low, this can take months but in the warmer environment of summer or a centrally heated house, this can be as short as a few days. The larvae feed on debris in the environment and, in warm conditions, rapidly develop into adult fleas to complete the life cycle. The dog flea is a different species to

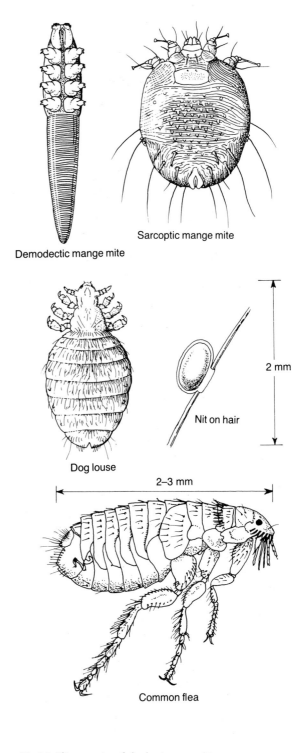

Demodectic mange mite

Sarcoptic mange mite

Dog louse

Nit on hair

2 mm

2–3 mm

Common flea

Fig 20 Skin parasites of the dog (not to scale)

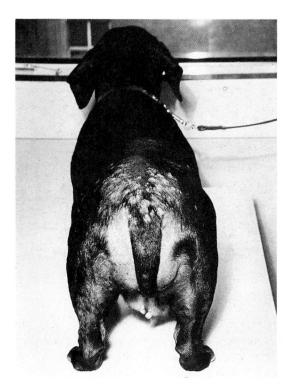

A typical case of flea dermatitis in a Smooth-Haired Dachshund.

the cat flea but a large proportion of fleas found on the dog are cat fleas. During a feed, a flea bites the skin of a dog and injects saliva into the skin to stop the blood from clotting. It then sucks up some blood, digests it and passes it out later on as small, shiny, black droppings. This flea dirt appears as little particles between the hairs of the dog's coat.

Fleas can affect dogs in two ways:

1 The dog becomes infested with fleas from other dogs or cats or his environment and becomes irritated by the mere presence of the fleas which are biting him. He will generally be itchy, especially in the summer months and fleas will be seen as reddish black, small, rapidly moving, side to side flattened insects, 3mm long, moving rapidly over the skin between the hairs.

2 A much more serious problem occurs if a dog becomes hypersensitive to, or allergic to, the flea saliva due to repeated exposure to flea bites. In this case, merely one bite every few days will render the dog permanently itchy and ensure that he scratches sufficiently to inflame the skin and lose hair over widespread areas, especially over his back and towards the base of his tail.

Diagnosis This is often straightforward. It is based on the type of lesions, the area affected, and the presence of fleas or flea droppings. If the particles seen are thought to be flea dirt, a useful test is to place some on a damp white tissue when flea dirt will soften and turn red within a short period as it is merely dried blood. The presence of one positive dropping on a dog who shows the characteristic lesions along the back, is enough to make a tentative diagnosis of flea allergic dermatitis despite the frequently encountered retort 'my dog has never had a flea!' They are extremely common and their presence does not indicate a dirty house – rather a pleasant, warm environment with deep pile carpet which is very attractive to fleas.

Treatment There is a whole range of parasiticidal preparations available to kill the fleas and any residual activity in the coat. Sprays and washes are far more effective than flea collars or powders and it is advisable to contact your vet to ascertain which product to use. Treatment must be continued on a regular basis, according to the manufacturer's instructions. In severe cases, it will be necessary for the vet to reduce the inflammation with drugs in the initial stages of treatment.

As the flea breeds in the environment around the house, it is advisable to treat any area in which the dog has been with a different type of insecticide to prevent eggs and larvae developing into adult fleas. Preparations are available from your vet.

It is worth mentioning here that both the dog and cat flea act as an intermediate host to the *Dipylidium* tapeworm. The flea larvae will eat tapeworm eggs that are deposited in the environment when the mature tapeworm segment dries and ruptures, scattering the eggs around. The egg develops into a cyst inside the flea and remains dormant until the adult flea irritates a dog which in biting itself, swallows the flea. The cyst is then released and develops into an adult tapeworm in the dog. Thus, routine tapeworm treatment should be considered in any dog which is shown to have a flea infestation.

Dog fleas will bite humans and may cause intense irritation. This is especially so on return from holiday to an empty house where the developing fleas have had no chance to feed for a few weeks as the dog has been to a boarding kennels. Numerous flea bites may appear around the ankles and the fleas may themselves be seen.

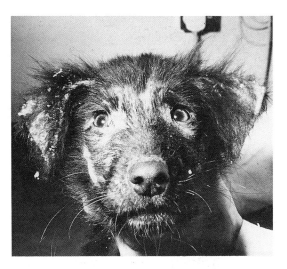

Sarcoptic mange in a mongrel puppy.

Lice

Dog lice are not seen as commonly as fleas and seem to occur more frequently in puppies and on the long-coated dogs. They can be seen with the naked eye as small, white or pale orange dots crawling very slowly between and up the hairs. The white single egg is attached to the hair and is known as a nit.

Lice do not cause a serious skin problem but, if present in sufficient numbers, they can produce small, itchy, scabby areas of eczema.

Diagnosis The presence of the lice themselves, or their eggs is considered diagnostic in an itchy dog. A hand lens may be useful to see them.

Treatment Modern parasiticidal preparations will kill the lice effectively and must be repeated at five- to seven-day intervals

until all the eggs have hatched. As the parasite completes its life cycle entirely on the dog, the environment does not have to be treated.

Sarcoptic Mange

This mange mite causes intense irritation by burrowing through the skin but, unlike the flea, it spends its entire life on the dog. Sarcoptic mange is very contagious and occurs more commonly in young dogs (*see* Chapter 4, page 56).

Rabbit Fur Mite (Cheyletiella)

As the name suggests, this mite lives mainly on the rabbit but it will infect dogs. It lives on the surface of the skin especially along the back. The irritation causes excessive dandruff formation.

Diagnosis The mite is similar in size and appearance to a grain of salt and can be seen under a microscope or magnifying glass. The vet will often ask you to provide some brushings of the dog's coat and to do this stand the dog on a large sheet of newspaper

111

and groom him. Add any debris from the brush to this, seal all the debris into a paper envelope and then into a polythene bag.

Treatment Modern parasiticide washes are the most effective treatment and your veterinary surgeon will advise on the duration of treatment.

This parasite is highly contagious to humans who develop a rash on areas that have been in contact with the dog.

Harvest Mites (Trombiculids)

Harvest mite infestation occurs in the late summer, starting about the middle to late July. The little orange harvest mite larvae infect the feet, legs and skin of the belly where they cause intense irritation.

Diagnosis The orange mites can just be seen with the naked eye or a hand lens on the legs especially. Any skin irritation which regularly develops in the late summer or early autumn on a dog is likely to be caused by these mites.

Treatment Modern, parasiticidal washes are the best treatment and your vet will advise on the duration of treatment.

Bacterial Infections (Pyoderma)

Bacterial skin infections are common in the dog and are usually secondary to some other skin disease, such as mange or allergies.

Folliculitis

This is a disease of the very short-coated breeds such as the Boxer, Dobermann and Pointers. The disease consists of multiple small pustules, usually on the muzzle, often on the feet, and sometimes on the back. The dog may appear to have numerous small clumps of raised hairs.

Treatment In mild cases, cleansing washes may be all that are required. In severe cases, a long course of antibiotics will be prescribed using an antibiotic that is identified by your vet from a skin swab. The condition is more common in the young dog and will often recur.

Impetigo

This is a common condition, especially, in our experience, in the Spaniel and Sheltie. The infection consists of rings of infection, mainly on the back and belly. These rings are inflamed and become hairless, and they may become crusted. As one lesion heals, another will often form.

Treatment Antibiotics identified from swabs and medicated shampoos are required but the disease frequently recurs.

Acute Moist Dermatitis (Wet Eczema)

This is a localised wet, painful, acute inflammation of the skin caused by excessive scratching or licking by the dog. It is seen more commonly in the Golden Retriever and German Shepherd. In the German Shepherd it often occurs on the rump and the initial irritation is thought to be impaction of the anal glands, although fleas are a possibility. In the Retriever, it usually occurs under the ear or on the side of the face. The initial cause is not fully understood but it is thought to be a secondary reaction to flea bites. If left untreated, the inflamed area can quickly become quite extensive.

Treatment The first stage of treatment is to clip away all the matted hair and clean the skin thoroughly to remove all discharge. The irritation must be reduced to lessen self trauma using anti-inflammatory creams and possibly injections, and antibiotics are usually

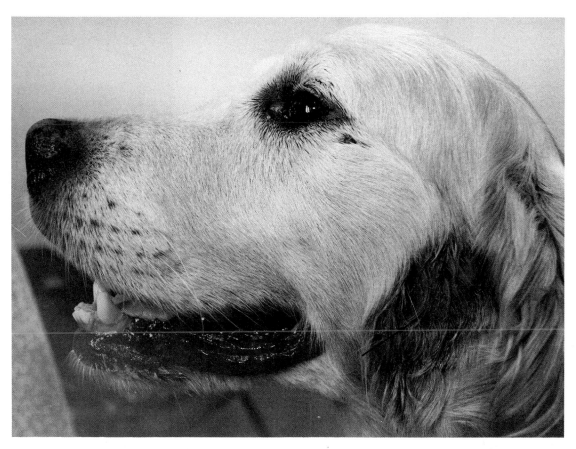

Wet eczema in a Golden Retriever.

necessary to clear up the infection. Any underlying cause such as impacted anal glands or fleas must also be treated. In the authors' experience, this condition clears more quickly if topical treatment of the lesion itself is avoided.

Skin Fold Pyoderma

Deep skin folds, such as those on the lower lips of Spaniels and Setters, or all over the body of Shar Peis, facial folds in Bulldogs and Pekes and deep folds around the vulva in overweight bitches are areas that are susceptible to bacterial infection. The fold becomes moist, inflamed and often very malodorous. It is often the smell which first draws the owner's attention to the lesion.

Treatment This consists of thoroughly cleansing and drying the infected skin and then applying an antibiotic/anti-inflammatory ointment. However, the disease is always likely to recur and surgery may be required to remove the excess skin which forms the fold.

Allergic Skin Disease

Contact Allergy

In this condition, the dog's skin becomes directly sensitised to some material in his environment such as wool, nylon, carpets or certain plants. The range of possible allergic substances is vast. The skin areas affected are usually on the underside of the body where the protective hair is thinnest, such as the belly, groin, axilla (armpit) and under-side of neck, chin or on the feet between the pads.

Initially, the skin becomes reddened but as the dog scratches it may develop a secondary infection. In long standing cases the skin becomes thickened and pigmented, due to the constant inflammation of the affected skin.

Treatment The ideal treatment would be to remove the allergic substance from the dog's environment. Skin testing is difficult in the dog, so your vet may suggest changing the dog's bedding, or taking the dog for a walk in a different area to try to find the cause. If this fails, then the irritation can be reduced by the use of anti-inflammatory creams, tablets or injections.

A useful diagnostic aid is to remove the dog from his normal environment for a few weeks, perhaps, to a friend's house or boarding kennels, when the problem may clear up spontaneously. If this happens, the cause of the allergy must be in the owner's home. The problem then arises in trying to identify the allergenic material.

Food Allergies

Food allergies are not very common in the dog, but when they occur, the affected dog will be itchy, generally all over his body. These skin symptoms may be accompanied by digestive upsets also. The three most common food allergies involve beef, milk and wheat.

Treatment If a food allergy is suspected, the dog should be fed on a diet of mutton and rice or a special commercial prescription diet for at least three weeks. If the skin irritation disappears following this test diet, then the dog's diet must be modified on a permanent basis.

Atopy

Atopy is a term used to describe an allergic reaction to an inhaled substance such as pollen. In man, atopy produces hay fever, while in the dog, atopy produces an itchy skin. The disease usually starts in the young dog in early summer when the pollen count is high and then the irritation drops away in the autumn. The dog simply becomes itchy, with very little to see on the surface of the skin except a slight inflammation. Later there will be hair loss and infection caused by the dog scratching and biting himself.

As the dog grows older, he may become itchy for a longer period each year. This is because gradually he becomes allergic to more substances until eventually he may scratch the whole year round.

Treatment As with contact dermatitis, it is very difficult to identify or eliminate the cause and most cases are treated with anti-inflammatory drugs. Antihistamine drugs are not so effective in the dog as they are in man.

Urticaria

This is an acute allergy in which the eyelids, nose and lips become swollen within a very short space of time. There may also be raised blotchy patches on the rest of the body. The cause is usually unknown and the condition normally responds to a single injection of an antihistamine or anti-inflammatory drugs. It tends not to be a recurring disease.

Other Itchy Skin Diseases
Auto-Immune Disease

An auto-immune disease occurs when, for some unknown reason, the dog's own defence mechanisms start to attack his own tissue. This can occur in the skin as well as

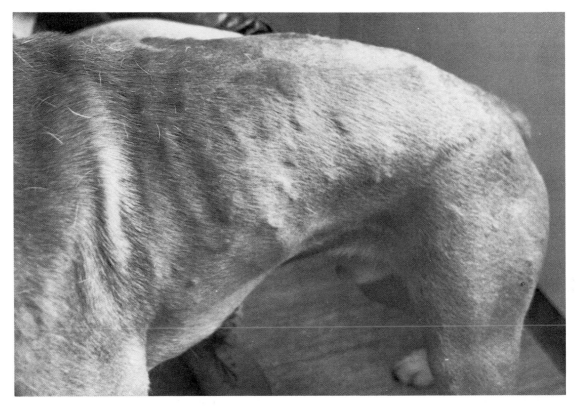

Widespread urticaria in a Boxer.

other tissues. Changes usually occur around the mouth, nose, eyes and anus. The skin becomes very inflamed and blisters or ulcers may form.

Diagnosis　The disease is diagnosed with the help of a skin biopsy.

Treatment　High levels of prednisolone, a corticosteroid, are required to suppress the disease and it may be necessary to continue them for a prolonged period, even years. In some cases, the disease is hard to control and extremely debilitating for the affected individual.

Contact Dermatitis

The symptoms and areas affected are identical to those of contact allergy but in this case the cause is a direct irritant.

Chemicals such as oil, disinfectant and detergents have been implicated.

Treatment　Anti-inflammatory creams and removal of the cause of the irritation usually rapidly reverse the dermatitis.

Lick Granuloma

Lick granulomas develop as raised, thickened, hairless patches of skin over the front of the carpus or the side of the hock. They are seen most commonly in the Labrador and develop there because the dog licks constantly at this one area. The underlying cause of this licking may be related to trauma, boredom or neurosis. The lesions are not harmful.

Treatment　These lesions are very difficult to treat because the constant licking develops

115

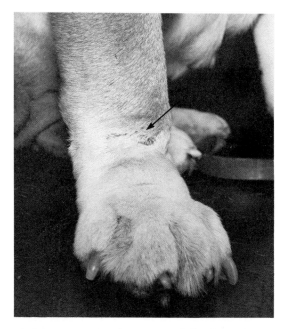

A lick granuloma of the right carpus of a bulldog.

into a habit. Anti-inflammatory creams, covering the lesion, surgical removal and cryosurgery are all used but with limited success.

Elbow Callus

Large heavy breeds such as St Bernards or Great Danes may develop a callus on one or both elbows. This is due to the sheer weight of the dog when he lies down, pressing the skin against the underlying bone. If untreated, a callus may become very inflamed and infected, and cause lameness.

Treatment A non-infected callus can be treated by applying surgical spirit to it on a daily basis on some cotton wool. This dries and toughens the skin.

An infected callus may require an antibiotic and a soft dressing. In some cases your vet may need to drain the infected callus surgically.

In all cases, a very soft bed should be provided for an affected dog.

NON-ITCHY SKIN DISEASES

Ticks

Ticks are found on dogs, especially in the summer months, and are usually parasites of sheep and cattle. The adult tick, initially small and spider-like, crawls over the body, finds a suitable place and bites into the skin. It now remains in this one spot for up to two weeks, engorges with blood and swells until it is the size of a pea. At this stage, it is usually beige or reddish in colour. It will now drop off and, if female, lay eggs in the grass. These hatch into larvae which similarly become attached to a passing host which may be a sheep, cow, dog, cat, rodent or man. After a feed, this larva drops off, undergoes change and finds another host. After these three larval stages, each one taking a year, the adult form is reached and the cycle recommences. This is the method by which sheep ticks are brought into the parks and verges of cities.

Treatment Ticks appear to cause very little irritation and are usually found by the owner during grooming. There are several ways in which the tick can be removed. It can be pulled off with fine forceps which grasp the tick where it is attached to the skin or it can be killed with cotton wool soaked in spirit or a parasiticide and then removed as above. Occasionally, the bite wound will become infected and need treatment. In some countries, ticks are the carriers of disease, such as Tick Borne Fever and Heartworm. Tick infestation can be prevented by the application of a modern parasiticide before taking the dog for a walk in the country.

Demodectic mange

As this disease is normally seen in young growing dogs, it is discussed in detail in Chapter 4 (*see* page 57).

Fungal Infections (Ringworm)

Ringworm is not very common in the dog and develops when the hairs and skin become invaded by the ringworm fungus. The hairs become weak and break off at the level of the skin, leaving bald patches. Ringworm can be caused by a fungus called *Microsporum canis* which in our experience is the most common ringworm found in dogs. Infected cats are often a source of this infection for the dog, and both species can also pass the infection on to man.

Another type of fungus, called *Trichophyton*, can also cause ringworm in the dog. Various species of this fungus affect cattle, horses, hedgehogs and rodents, all of which can transmit the infection to inquisitive dogs. *Trichophyton* can also be transmitted from all species to man.

Ringworm usually starts to develop on the face or forelegs, as single or multiple areas of hair loss. As the disease progresses, these areas can become quite large and may become infected, producing a purulent sore. In the early stages, the affected skin assumes the appearance of cigarette ash.

Diagnosis The majority of ringworm infections caused by *Microsporum* will fluoresce a lime green colour in the dark under an ultraviolet light called a 'Wood's lamp'. This test is usually diagnostic, but if the suspected lesion fails to fluoresce, or if confirmation is advisable, hair samples can be examined and cultured in a laboratory. Microscopic examination may be diagnostic but if not, as the fungus takes time to grow, the result will not be available for two to three weeks. It is important to ascertain whether the disease is definitely ringworm because of the risk of transfer to people.

Treatment When handling dogs with ringworm, the owners must be very careful and should wear rubber gloves. The area surrounding the lesion should be clipped to remove as much infected hair as possible and the skin thoroughly cleaned with a fungicidal wash. These clippings should be burnt. In mild cases fungicidal ointment or lotion may eliminate the lesions but usually an antibiotic called griseofulvin which kills the fungus, is given in tablet form for between four and eight weeks. Further brushings of the coat may be examined at this stage to see if any fungus remains and an examination with the Wood's lamp every two weeks or so will provide an assessment of the success of treatment.

Hormonal Skin Disease

Dogs with fine feathering such as spaniels, retrievers and Afghans may develop a more woolly-looking coat after neutering. This is not harmful but many owners feel that it spoils the dog's good looks so this may be a contraindication to neutering.

Hormonal hair loss is an uncommon skin complaint but appears to be more common in the very short-coated breeds, such as the Dobermann and Boxer. The hair loss usually starts on the flanks, and is not normally accompanied by itching or infection. Several different hormones, e.g. thyroid and sex hormones, may be implicated and laboratory testing of a blood sample is required to identify the cause. Specific hormone replacement therapy can then be instigated.

There are two specific hormonal diseases which will cause hair loss as part of the disease process.

Cushing's Disease

The adrenal glands become over-active and produce an excessive amount of steroids. This slowly results in an overweight dog who has an excessive appetite and thirst. He becomes lethargic, his muscles weaken, and his skin thins and shows extensive hair loss, mainly on the trunk.

Treatment Cushing's disease is diagnosed in the laboratory from blood samples. The disease can be treated by the surgical removal of the adrenal glands and replacement hormone therapy or sometimes by tablets which suppress adrenal function.

Sertoli Cell Tumours

These occur in the testicles of male dogs, especially in those testicles which have not descended into the scrotal sac. They produce excessive amounts of female hormones which cause the dog to undergo feminisation, with mammary development, shrinkage of the male sex organs and hair loss, again mainly on the body.

Treatment The clinical signs in a male dog and the enlargement of a testicle are diagnostic. The signs are reversible when the enlarged testicle is removed surgically.

TUMOURS AND CYSTS

Sebaceous Cysts

These are often felt as round painless nodules in the skin and vary from a match-head to a plum in size. They are seen commonly in German Shepherd Dogs, Shelties and Pekes and are a recurring problem. Sometimes, these cysts will rupture and release a thick white secretion. If, at this stage, they are bathed in saline and all the material is removed, they may heal spontaneously. However, if they become infected, surgical excision may be necessary.

Warts

Warts are very common in the older dog, especially in breeds such as Spaniels and Poodles. Some patients have a great number of warts but they very rarely cause problems.

Occasionally, a dog will persistently chew or damage a wart causing haemorrhage and in such a case surgical excision is the treatment of choice.

Tumours

Skin tumours are commonly found in the dog. Most are benign but some are malignant and spread or regrow after surgical excision. If left untreated they can become quite large, and if on the underside of the body may interfere with walking. Sometimes the surface of a large tumour may ulcerate and become infected, forming an unpleasant sore.

Treatment In most cases, it is impossible for the vet to differentiate skin tumours by their appearance and therefore, surgical removal at an early stage is advisable in order to reduce the possibility of recurrence or spread. An analysis of the tumour at a laboratory will identify the tumour and

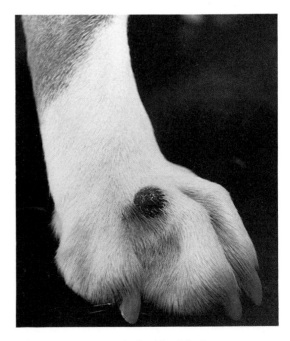

A histiocytoma tumour in the skin of the foot.

enable an assessment to be made of the chances of recurrence.

DISEASES OF THE ANAL AREA

Anal Adenoma

In the old male dog tumours, called anal adenomas, frequently develop around the anus. These tumours are very vascular and ulcerate when they are still quite small to produce small bleeding points.

Treatment Anal adenomas will sometimes regress if the dog is treated with large doses of the female hormone, stilboestrol, or if he is castrated. In other cases, surgical removal is necessary.

Anal Sac Impaction

This is very common in the dog and all breeds are affected. However, in our experience, the smaller breeds such as the Cavalier King Charles Spaniel and Miniature Poodle are more frequently affected. The anal sac secretion slowly accumulates in the gland instead of being expressed during defaecation, the impacted anal sacs become itchy and sore and the dog will drag his anus along the ground or bite himself around the base of his tail.

The full glands can be felt through the skin below the anus and are emptied by the vet using manual pressure. The anal sac material is constantly being produced and the frequency with which the glands refill is variable. In some dogs it can be as rapid as two weeks.

Treatment In mild infrequent cases, it is sufficient to empty the anal sacs when necessary. Where the problem is recurrent, surgical removal of the anal sacs is necessary.

Anal Abscess

Occasionally, an impacted gland will become infected to form an abscess. Usually, only one gland is affected, but the condition is very painful and the dog may be depressed and off his food. The abscess usually discharges through the skin over the area of the anal sac.

Treatment The infected gland should be bathed and cleaned, and excess pus removed. A short course of antibiotics may be necessary, either given in tablet or injection form, or by ointment instilled into the gland. Very occasionally, infections will affect the same sacs repeatedly and surgical excision will be necessary.

Anal Furunculosis

This is a painful skin disease, characterised by raw, discharging sinuses and cavities in the skin around the anus. It is almost always

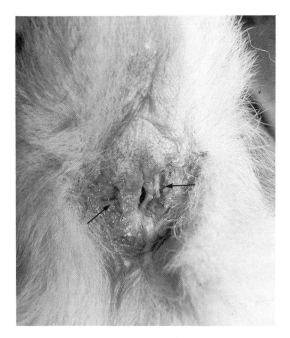

Severe anal furunculosis in a German Shepherd Dog.

119

confined to the German Shepherd Dog and is thought to be connected with the way his bushy tail is held low over the anus. It is postulated that infection spreads from the anal sac into the surrounding humid areas which then develop these discharging wounds. If left untreated, the whole area can become devoid of skin. It is a very painful disease.

Treatment Antibiotic treatment may give temporary respite but we believe that surgery to remove the infected tissue and anal glands should be instigated as soon as possible. This is normally successful and usually a combination of conventional surgery and cryosurgery (freezing) is used. However, the removal of an extensive area of infection may result in severe scarring around the anus, causing constipation or faecal incontinence.

Furunculosis can occur elsewhere on the body, especially in the skin of the elbows and hocks of the larger breeds. Discharging sinuses are seen and treatment may again involve surgery.

DISEASES OF THE FEET

Interdigital Eczema

Dogs will readily lick their feet following minor damage such as grazes, bruises or thorn damage. This licking makes the feet very wet especially in breeds with heavy feathering, and this in turn leads to infection of the feet between the pads. The infection causes pain and so the dog continues to lick at his feet setting up a vicious circle of events. Lameness invariably results.

Treatment The foot must be cleaned, the excess hair clipped away and a search made for thorns. The foot should be dried and bandaged for five to seven days to prevent further licking. Anti-inflammatory and antibiotic creams will help to reduce the inflammation.

Interdigital Cysts and Abscesses

Painful swellings occur between the toes in a variety of breeds. They may be very large and make the dog very lame. Cysts will often burst spontaneously and then regress for a while only to develop again. They can be frustrating to treat because even after extensive surgery they will often return. In most cases the cause is unknown but some breeds, such as the Bull Terrier and Dobermann, have narrow spaces between the toes which can occasionally lead to interdigital problems due to friction.

Treatment Lancing of the cyst and frequent bathing in warm saline will provide immediate relief of pain. Antibiotics, antiinflammatory drugs and surgery are all used in the treatment of these cysts with mixed results.

Foreign Body Cysts

These can easily be mistaken for interdigital cysts. The most common cause is the penetration of the skin between the toes by a grass seed, especially in the hairy breeds, such as Spaniels and Old English Sheepdogs. This problem usually occurs in late summer. The dog develops a painful discharging swelling between the toes and if the grass seed is not removed it will move up the leg under the skin.

Treatment If the seed can be seen it should be gently but completely pulled out. Once it has penetrated through the skin, probing with forceps may locate and remove it but, if not, surgery should be carried out as soon as possible, before the seed has a chance to move.

Foreign Bodies in the Pads

The most common foreign bodies are sharp spicules of glass or thorns but even these are remarkably rare as the surface of the pad is very tough. The dog is usually very lame and the affected pad painful with a small opening on the surface. Pressure on the pad will increase the pain.

Treatment A general anaesthetic may be needed to enlarge the opening to enable removal of the glass fragment or thorn but occasionally it is possible to remove them by digital pressure.

Broken Nails

Dogs frequently break their claws especially if they are too long. This can be very painful and draws the owner's attention to the problem. If the break does not affect the nail bed, the broken portion can simply be clipped away but if the nail bed or quick is involved, it will usually be necessary to remove the nail under an anaesthetic. Most nails will re-grow normally in time.

Nail Bed Infections

Infection can enter the tip of a toe through a damaged nail bed. The tip becomes swollen and painful and the dog lame. Such infections are usually treated with a long course of a suitable antibiotic but, if neglected, the small bones may become diseased, the joints arthritic and this can lead to amputation of the affected toe.

Fungal Infection of the Nail Bed

This is a rare infection of the nail which becomes loose and easily shed. The infection is diagnosed by culturing the fungus from an infected nail in a laboratory. Long-term fungicidal treatment is necessary.

Overgrown Nails

Most dogs fortunately do not require regular nail clipping as the nails wear down naturally during exercise. Older dogs, or those from smaller breeds can develop very long claws which require cutting on a regular basis. An easy test to ascertain whether your dog's nails are too long is to stand the dog on a flat surface and if the nails touch the ground they are too long. White nails are easier to clip as the pink quick can be seen. The nail should be cut about 3mm ($\frac{1}{10}$in) nearer the tip than the quick. Black nails, however, are more difficult and should be left to the expert. Occasionally, a nail, especially on the dew claw, will grow in a circle and penetrate the dog's pad. The pad will become infected and painful. The answer is to cut the nail and bathe the sore in saline. Sometimes, if the infection is severe, antibiotics may be needed. If this becomes a recurring problem the dew claw can be removed.

10 The Ear

The ear has two separate functions. One function is to receive sound waves and convert these into messages which are passed to the brain, and the other is to appreciate movement and balance so that the dog is aware of his position in relation to the ground.

NORMAL STRUCTURE AND FUNCTION

The ear can be divided into three distinct parts:

The outer ear This consists of the ear flap, or pinna, which continues as the external ear canal and ends at the ear-drum. The pinna is composed of a layer of cartilage covered on both sides by skin. Its function is to trap sound waves and so its

natural position is erect. However, in many breeds the pinna now folds over the entrance to the ear canal.

The ear canal is an L-shaped tube with a horizontal and a vertical portion. It is composed of cartilage which is covered by a special skin, containing wax-secreting glands. The ear-drum is a thin round membrane across the canal which vibrates when stimulated by sound waves. The ear canal is normally free of hair but in some breeds such as Poodles, hair is present. Some individuals have excessively hairy canals, and the implications of this are discussed later (*see* page 125).

The middle ear The middle and inner ear are enclosed within bone at the base of the skull. The middle ear is an air-filled cavity which is connected to the throat by a fine tube, the eustachian tube. Sound waves

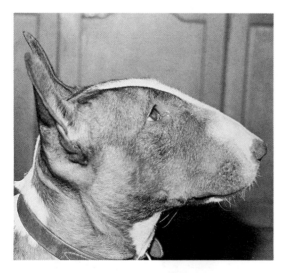

This Bull Terrier shows well-ventilated 'prick' ears.

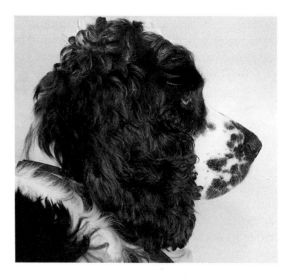

This spaniel shows poorly ventilated 'flop' ears.

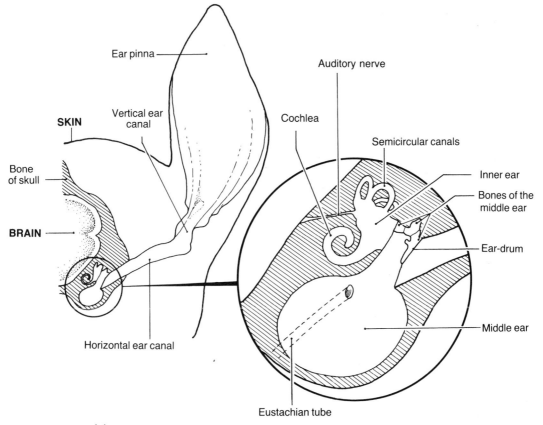

Fig 21 Structure of the ear

are transmitted from the ear-drum across the middle ear by three small bones to another small membrane which separates the middle and inner ear.

The inner ear   The inner ear is composed of a number of small fluid-filled tubes. One of these, the cochlea, converts the sound vibrations into messages which pass along the auditory nerve to the brain. The semi-circular canals are arranged on either side of the skull so that any movement of the head sets up a disturbance in the fluid. This disturbance is monitored by little hair-like sensors at the end of the auditory nerve which gives the dog its sense of balance.

DISEASES OF THE EAR PINNA

The ear pinna is very susceptible to damage. It has a large blood supply, so wounds will often bleed profusely. By violently shaking his ear, the dog will splatter the surrounding area with specks of blood. It is often necessary to suture even the smallest of wounds to stop further haemorrhage.

Short-coated dogs who persistently shake their head can split the tip of the pinna where it hits the head. If untreated, this damage is repaired by scar tissue which is weaker than normal skin. Therefore, the ear tip becomes more susceptible to damage from further head shaking. Once scar tissue has formed on the ear tip, little can be done to prevent further damage, except to ascertain the cause of head shaking and to correct this.

The ear pinna can often be more heavily infected with lice or sarcoptic mange than the rest of the body. These diseases are described in greater detail in Chapter 9 (*see* page 111).

Bilateral Hair Loss

In certain breeds, especially the Dachshund and Poodle, the ears can become quite hairless and the skin pigmented and leathery. This may be unsightly but it is not harmful to the dog. There is no treatment.

Haematoma

A haematoma is a painless, blood-filled swelling of the pinna caused by rupture of the blood vessels in the cartilage. Haematomas are caused either by a knock or by constant shaking of the ears due to an ear infection or irritation.

Treatment If untreated, the blood clot will slowly be replaced by scar tissue. As the scar tissue contracts, the pinna will be pulled out of shape which as well as being unsightly, may block the entrance to the ear canal. In man, this is often referred to as a cauliflower ear. To prevent this distortion of the ear, the blood clot can be removed surgically through an incision on the underside of the pinna. Sutures are then placed through the pinna to hold the two sides together and prevent any further accumulation of blood. The sutures are left in place for about two weeks.

DISEASES OF THE EAR CANAL

Infection (Otitis Externa)

This is a major problem in many breeds of dog. There are many causes of ear infection but one of the most important causes is

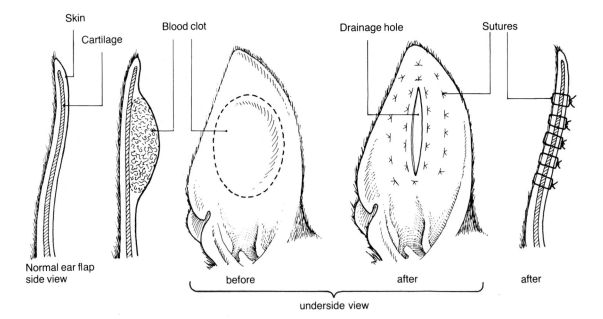

Skin
Cartilage
Blood clot
Drainage hole
Sutures

Normal ear flap side view

before

after

after

underside view

Fig 22 Aural haematoma before and after repair

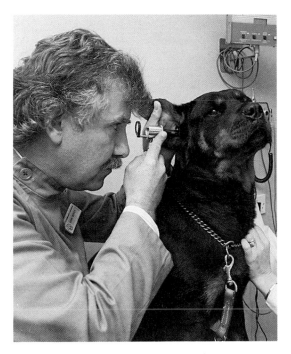

The auriscope in use in the examination of this Rottweiler's ear.

lack of adequate ventilation. This is seen most commonly in the hairy breeds in which the ear pinna is folded tightly against the head. Examples are the Cocker Spaniel, Golden Retriever and Old English Sheepdog. Some dogs have very narrow canals or excessive folding of the inside layers, both of which can lead to poor ventilation and, in some cases, ulceration of the folds. In some breeds, such as the Poodle, there is excessive hair growth in the canal, which retains wax, and this again reduces air flow. Many dogs with ear infections also have a concurrent skin infection but because of the factors mentioned above, the skin of the ear canal is particularly affected. Ear mites, and foreign bodies such as grass seeds will also produce an initial irritation which results in the buildup of wax. The accumulation of wax within the ear canal sets up an inflammation, which then becomes infected by various bacteria

and moulds. The canal becomes more inflamed with the accumulation of pus and further deposits of wax. If the infection is allowed to progress, the skin becomes thickened and the underlying cartilage becomes hard and calcified. This reduces the diameter of the canal even further, with a corresponding reduction in air flow and drainage of wax.

The clinical signs of otitis externa can vary greatly depending on the speed and severity of onset. In mild cases, there may be little to see apart from an increase in wax. As the disease progresses, the ear begins to smell, the discharge increases and the dog shakes his head, scratches his ear or rubs it along the ground. The ear may become very painful and the dog resents examination. Sometimes, however, the ear will become extremely inflamed very quickly, with pain and redness as the first signs of trouble.

Diagnosis   The diagnosis of an ear infection is normally straightforward. Your vet will examine the ear first with the naked eye and then with an auriscope (an instrument for looking in ears). Although sometimes uncomfortable for the dog, this is not normally painful and is usually carried out in the vet's consulting room. Sometimes, however, an anaesthetic may be necessary for a thorough investigation. This initial examination will often indicate the cause of the problem.

Treatment   The first stage of treatment is a thorough cleansing of the canal. The method used will depend on the nature of the dog and the amount of discharge. In a good-natured dog with little discharge, the instillation of drops may be sufficient, but it may be necessary to continue this for a few days. In more severe cases, the ears can be syringed under a general anaesthetic. Antibiotic, fungicidal and anti-inflammatory drugs may then be applied to kill the infection and reduce the inflammation.

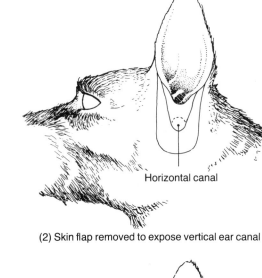

(1) Line of incision

line of skin incision

(2) Skin flap removed to expose vertical ear canal

Horizontal canal

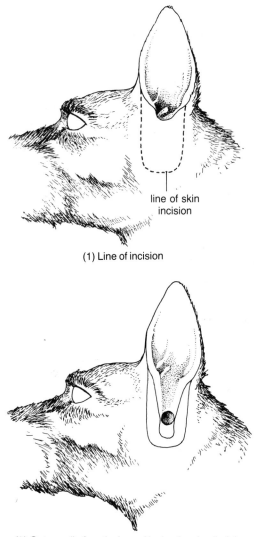

(3) Outer wall of vertical canal incised and pulled down

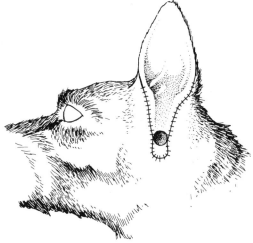

(4) Skin and ear canal sutured together

Fig 23 Aural resection operation

Laboratory testing of an ear swab will identify the infection and help in the choice of the correct antibiotic. Most ear infections will respond to this initial treatment, but recurrences are common. These can be minimised by vigilance on the part of the owner, early treatment or removal of wax, and the regular plucking of hairy ears.

Where recurring infections cause discomfort to the dog, surgery may be necessary. This will be of greatest benefit in cases that have not developed to the stage where the skin is thickened and the cartilage calcified. The aim of surgery is to increase the air flow to the canal and allow greater drainage of ear secretions. This is achieved by removing the outer wall of the vertical canal in an operation known as an aural resection. If the canal is grossly thickened and damaged then the vet will carry out a vertical canal ablation, in which the whole of the vertical canal is removed.

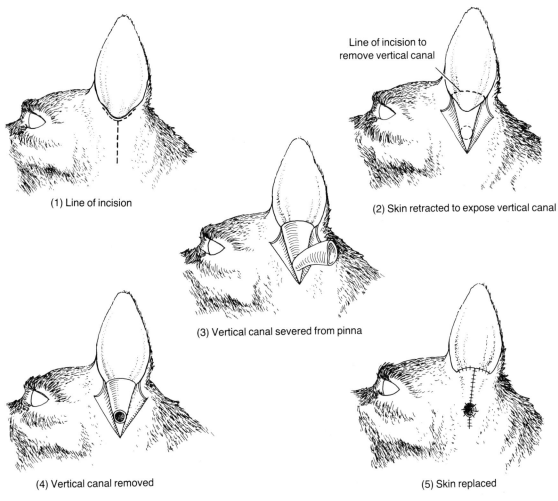

(1) Line of incision

Line of incision to remove vertical canal

(2) Skin retracted to expose vertical canal

(3) Vertical canal severed from pinna

(4) Vertical canal removed

(5) Skin replaced

Fig 24 *Vertical canal ablation operation*

The underlying causes of outer ear disease in the dog explain why otitis externa becomes a challenge for the vet, frustrating for the owner and, more importantly, a source of chronic irritation for the dog.

Ear mites

Ear mites are microscopic spider-like parasites which live in the ear canal of dogs and cats. They spread readily between the two species, the cat often being the source of the infection in dogs. Mite infestations are very common in young puppies, and are described

fully in Chapter 4, The Growing Dog (*see* page 59).

Foreign Bodies

Foreign objects are rarely found in dogs' ears, with the main exception of grass seeds which can become a considerable problem in late summer. These are seen mostly in breeds with hairy, floppy ears, especially the Cocker Spaniel. The grass seeds become trapped in the hair on the underside of the ear pinna and, because of their shape, they gradually work their way into and down

127

the ear canal until they lie against the ear-drum.

Diagnosis The usual history is that the dog has been for a walk in, or near long grass, and suddenly starts to shake his head violently. The grass seed can only be seen with the auriscope, but, because of the discomfort, the vet may have to examine him under sedation or a general anaesthetic.

Treatment Except in the quietest of dogs, removal of the seed is usually carried out under general anaesthesia, using long fine forceps through the auriscope.

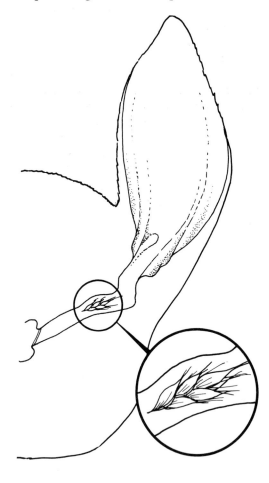

Fig 25 Grass seed in the ear, illustrating why it only moves one way

Tumours

Very occasionally a tumour or polyp will grow in the ear canal and gradually cause a blockage. Infection will develop and the symptoms will be similar to those of otitis externa. The tumour will normally be visible to the vet using an auriscope.

Treatment It is usually possible to remove the tumour surgically although it may be necessary to perform an aural resection to reach it.

DISEASES OF THE MIDDLE EAR

Infection (Otitis Media)

Infection of the middle ear normally develops from otitis externa through a damaged ear-drum, but occasionally it can reach the middle ear through the eustachian tube. As otitis media is nearly always associated with otitis externa, the symptoms are very similar – head shaking, rubbing the ear, head held to one side, pain and discharge.

Diagnosis Middle-ear disease can be diagnosed by careful examination of the ear-drum using the auriscope. A torn ear-drum will imply that infection has entered the middle-ear. In long-standing cases, the air-filled spaces become full of pus and the surrounding bone thickened and irregular. An X-ray of the skull will reveal these changes.

Treatment The treatment is similar to that of disease of the external canal. The ear is syringed to remove all discharge and then an ear preparation containing antibiotics, fungicidal and/or anti-inflammatory drugs is instilled. Again the underlying cause must be identified to prevent or minimise recurrence.

DISEASES OF THE INNER EAR

Infection (Otitis Interna)

The infection in middle-ear disease may spread directly to the inner ear. The symptoms will be similar to those of otitis externa and otitis media but the dog may also be deaf. However, as the inner ear also controls balance, inflammation of the semi-circular canals will produce a disturbance in the dog's posture. This is shown by a head tilt, walking in circles or falling over, all to the affected side. A flicking movement of the eyes, known as nystagmus, will also frequently be present.

Treatment   The treatment is again similar to that for otitis externa, although a course of antibiotic and anti-inflammatory injections or tablets are usually necessary in addition to ear drops or ointments.

DEAFNESS

There are no specific tests for deafness in the dog available to the general practitioner. To assess a dog's hearing it is necessary to study his response to noises of varying intensity. Total deafness in the younger dog is very uncommon and few puppies are born deaf. Large floppy ears and hairy ear canals must to a certain extent reduce keenness of hearing.

Severe otitis externa with thickening of the canal walls, blockage of the canal with discharge, or damage to the ear-drum will reduce hearing. Normal hearing will return with prompt treatment of the infection. Otitis interna may cause a severe impairment of hearing which can be permanent, despite treatment. The degree of loss of hearing will depend on the severity of the infection and whether one, or both, ears are affected.

Senile deafness is, however, common in dogs. As with man, hearing becomes less acute with age and care must be taken by owners not to lose contact with an older dog while he is away from familiar territory. A partially deaf dog will often retain the ability to hear a hand clap long after he can no longer hear the owner's voice. So as soon as senile deafness is suspected, it is wise to train him to recognise this sound.

11 The Eye

The eye has developed to receive light images from the dog's surroundings and to convert these images into nerve messages which can be passed to a special part of his brain, called the visual cortex.

NORMAL STRUCTURE AND FUNCTION

The eye works in a similar way to a camera. Light rays pass through the cornea, a clear window in the front of the eye, and through the pupil which is the black central circle in the middle of the eye. The amount of light entering the eye is controlled by the iris, which changes the diameter of the pupil. The iris is the coloured area around the pupil and in the dog it is usually brown.

Light rays are focused by the lens, which lies just behind the pupil, on to a light sensitive layer at the back of the eye, the retina. The retina then converts the light rays into nerve impulses which pass to the brain along the optic nerve. The part of the eye between the lens and the cornea is the anterior chamber and it is filled with a watery fluid, the aqueous, which is maintained at a constant pressure. The posterior chamber behind the lens is filled with a clear jelly-like material, the vitreous. The aqueous is constantly being produced in the eye and drained through an area at the base of the iris, called the drainage angle. This ensures that the fluid is always clean and healthy.

The eye is protected from behind by the skull and in front by the upper and lower

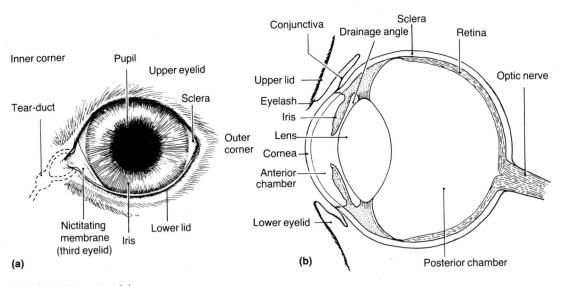

Fig 26 (a) Front view of the eye
(b) Section through the eye

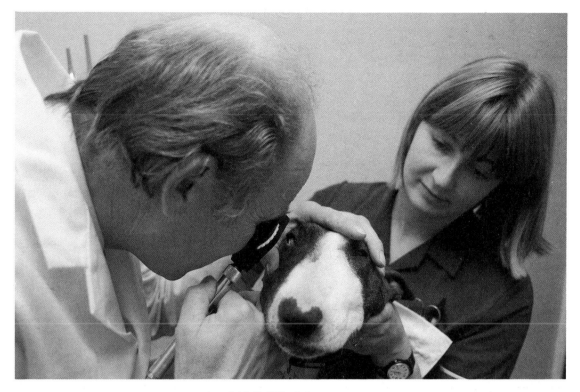

The ophthalmoscope in use in the examination of this Bull Terrier's eye.

eyelids. There is also a third eyelid, the nictitating membrane, situated at the inner corner of the eye which can be moved across to give further protection. The eyelids are lined by a membrane, the conjunctiva, and this continues on to the white surface of the eye, the sclera. Tears, constantly produced by small tear glands, ensure that the eye remains moist at all times. Excess tears are removed by two small tear ducts which start on the inner corner of the eyelids, run along the inside of the nose and discharge just inside each nostril. Each eye is moved from behind by six small muscles.

Dogs rely far less on vision for assessing their environment than other animals such as cats. Many dogs with poor eyesight cope very well and some are almost totally blind before there is any noticeable change in behaviour. There are few tests available in general practice to assess a dog's vision and

his loss of eyesight can be deduced only from the degree of damage to the various structures of the eye. Hair is impermeable to light and any dog whose hair is allowed to grow down over his eyes will have reduced vision. Breeds where this is likely to happen include the Old English Sheepdog, Bearded Collie and Tibetan Terrier.

Examination of the eye The instrument that the vet uses to examine the eye closely is called an ophthalmoscope. This is, in reality, a small torch which lights up the eye, incorporating a lens and focusing device so the vet can examine the whole depth of the eye from the cornea at the front to the retina at the back. It may be necessary for the vet to place drops in the dog's eyes to cause the pupils to widen as this will permit a more thorough examination of the eye.

131

DISEASES OF THE EYELIDS AND ASSOCIATED STRUCTURES

The edge of the eyelid must sit snugly against the eyeball as, if there is a gap, tears and dirt can accumulate and this may lead to infection. Wounds to the eyelids can cause deformity due to scarring and this may result in poor conformation of the eyelids. However, most cases of eyelid deformity are developmental and are seen in breeds with a lot of loose skin around the head such as the Cocker Spaniel, Bloodhound and especially the Shar Pei.

Entropion

In this condition, there is an in-rolling of the edge of the eyelid so that the lashes and hairs rub against the surface of the eye. Entropion can affect one or both eyes and upper or lower eyelids, and in severe cases, all four lids can be affected.

Entropion is usually a disease of the young, growing dog. It causes irritation and inflammation of the eyeball so the dog is reluctant to open the affected eye, which produces an excess of tears. If the condition is not treated, the constant rubbing of the hairs against the surface of the eye may produce ulceration of the cornea. This is a very serious complication and requires immediate treatment.

Occasionally, a severe primary infection of the eye will lead to spasm of the eyelids which then produces an in-rolling of the eyelid edge as a secondary effect.

Treatment This is essential and consists of the surgical removal of a small area of the outer surface of the eyelid which returns the lid margin to its normal position.

Ectropion

Ectropion is the opposite of entropion and here the edge of the eyelid droops away from the eye. It is less serious than entropion but gives rise to an unsightly inflamed eye.

Treatment Surgery is usually the treatment chosen but is not always as successful as that for entropion. Many surgical tech-

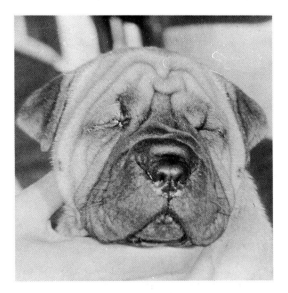

A Shar Pei puppy with entropion of all four eyelids.

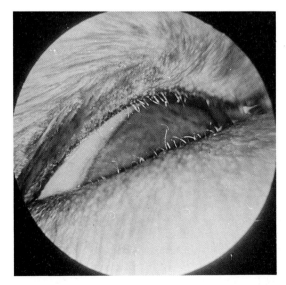

The eye of a Pekingese showing distichiasis.

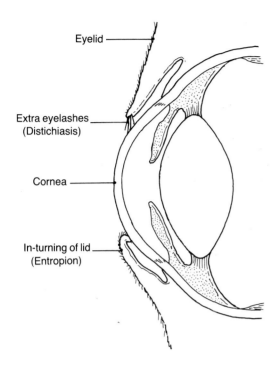

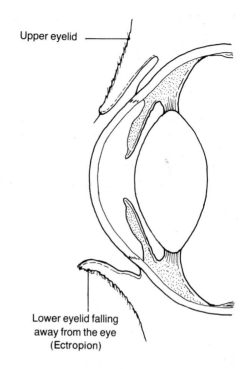

Eyelid

Extra eyelashes
(Distichiasis)

Cornea

In-turning of lid
(Entropion)

Upper eyelid

Lower eyelid falling
away from the eye
(Ectropion)

Fig 27 Entropion, ectropion and distichiasis

niques are available but although the condition is usually improved, it is not always eliminated.

In some breeds, such as the Dobermann and Rough Collie, a small area of the lower lid in the inner corner does not always sit tightly against the eye. Although this does not cause any serious problems, owners often notice a buildup of mucus in this area, especially after the dog has been sleeping. No treatment is necessary and this mucus should be simply wiped away.

Distichiasis

In this condition, fine hairs grow along the very edge of the eyelid and rub against the cornea. This constant rubbing irritates the eye and leads to excessive tear production which wets the area around the eye.

Treatment This is aimed at removing the extra malpositioned hairs and the following techniques are available to your vet.

1 Each individual hair can be plucked out by the vet who may need to use a lens to visualise them as they are so fine. As lashes so removed will always re-grow, the owner may be able to learn how to carry out this procedure gently.
2 Each individual hair can be removed by electrolysis.
3 A wedge section of the entire length of the edge of the eyelid, including the hair roots, can be surgically removed.

Infection (Periorbital Dermatitis)

The skin of the eyelids is very thin and occasionally susceptible to infection, which is usually associated with conjunctivitis.

The eyelids will be inflamed, painful, swollen and often moist with scab formation. An overflow of tears in the inner corner of the eye will produce a localised infection of the skin of this area.

Treatment Periorbital dermatitis is treated by cleaning the eyelids with warm, sterile water and cotton wool, and then applying an ointment containing antibiotics and often anti-inflammatory drugs. Some ointments can be placed in the eye as well as on the eyelids, but before doing this, it is wise to check with the vet. Any underlying cause, such as entropion, atopy or demodex, must also be corrected.

Non-Function of Tear-Ducts

Blockage of the tear-ducts will lead to an overflow of tears from the inner corner of the eye. This leads to tear staining on one or both sides of the nose and this is most obvious in white-faced dogs. Dogs may be born with small, or absent, tear-duct openings. This condition is seen most commonly in the Cocker Spaniel. Ducts may become blocked with pus or mucus during eye infections. Dogs with very short muzzles may have narrow tear-ducts with a corresponding delay in drainage.

Blocked tear-ducts are diagnosed by placing a drop of a dye called fluorescein onto the surface of the eye. Green drops will appear at the nostrils within a few minutes in dogs with normal tear-ducts but failure of this dye to appear on either side shows that there is a blockage in the corresponding duct.

Treatment This is carried out under a general anaesthetic as the openings of the ducts are very small and difficult to locate. If the duct openings are absent, very little can be done. If the opening is present, a very fine canula is inserted and the duct is flushed out with sterile saline.

Prolapse of the Harderian Gland

Behind the nictitating membrane is a small, fleshy mass of pink tissue called the Harderian gland whose function is to help remove infection from the eye. In some young dogs, especially the Shih Tzu and American Cocker Spaniel, it can become displaced and be seen protruding from behind the nictitating membrane. This prolapsed gland is unsightly, irritates the eye and causes excessive tear production.

Treatment Surgical removal or replacement is necessary and this is a minor procedure, which has no adverse effect on the eye. General anaesthesia is, however, necessary.

Eversion of the Nictitating Membrane

Occasionally in young dogs, especially in our experience German Shepherds, the edge of the nictitating membrane rolls outwards and folds over on itself. It is usually seen in the young puppy and it is unsightly, may irritate the eye and cause excessive tear production.

Treatment The small portion of rolled tissue is removed surgically under a general anaesthetic.

Prolapse of the Eye

(*See also* Chapter 18, page 220). The eye can be forced out of its bony orbit in one of two ways:

Trauma

A severe blow to the head caused by, for instance, a road traffic accident or a fight with another dog, may force the eye out of its socket. This type of injury is more common in the large-eyed, short-nosed dog, such as the Pekingese, where the orbit of the eye is shallow.

Treatment To prevent permanent damage, the eye must be replaced immediately under a general anaesthetic. Sometimes, because of damage within the orbit, such as a fractured bone or massive haemorrhage, it is not possible to replace the eye and surgical removal will be necessary.

A Mass within the Eye Socket

Any swelling behind the eye will slowly push it forward making it more prominent and, therefore, difficult for the dog to close his eyelids. The two most common causes are abscesses and tumours.

Treatment Abscesses will often respond to antibiotics and the eye will return to its normal position.

Tumours in the orbit are not easy to treat and removal of the eye may be necessary to reach the tumour. Many are malignant and surgery may be impossible or of no benefit to the dog.

Horner's Syndrome

This is an uncommon condition in which the small autonomic nerves to the eye are damaged. The cause is usually difficult to establish and may involve trauma to the neck or middle ear disease. The symptoms are drooping of the upper eyelid, prominence of the third eyelid and constriction of the iris. Vision is unimpaired. (*See also* Chapter 13, page 173).

Nystagmus

This is a rapid, spontaneous movement of both eyes which is caused by damage to the part of the brain which controls balance. The movement consists of a fast flicker of the eye to the affected side with a slow return to its resting position. (*See also* Vestibular Syndrome in Chapter 13, page 165).

Tumours

Small wart-like growths are seen frequently on the eyelid margins of old dogs. These small tumours will rub against the eyeball and cause irritation.

Treatment Provided they are not allowed to grow too big, the tumours can be removed surgically by a small wedge-shaped resection of the eyelid to ensure the 'roots' are included.

DISEASES OF THE CONJUNCTIVA

Conjunctivitis

Conjunctivitis, or inflammation of the conjunctiva, is common in the dog and causes the white of the eye to appear red. It can vary from mild to very severe. Where a mild conjunctivitis is present, symptoms may be few, perhaps a slight redness and irritation with increased tear production. However, in severe conjunctivitis the eye is very painful and red, and the eyelids may be closed (blepharospasm). There will be a profuse discharge which may vary from watery to a thick, grey/green pus, and the dog will resent having his eye examined.

Possible causes of conjunctivitis include viruses, especially canine distemper virus, bacteria, chemicals, allergies, trauma or foreign bodies.

The vet will examine the eye very carefully to ascertain the cause. Usually, if one eye only is affected, the cause is local to that eye but if both are involved, the conjunctivitis may be part of a general disease process.

Treatment The eyes must be bathed with warm sterile water and, depending on the case, treated with antibiotic and/or anti-inflammatory drops or ointment. Most cases of conjunctivitis respond to treatment but laboratory tests may be necessary to ascertain the cause, and correct line of treatment.

Sometimes the occurrence of conjunctivitis is a reflection of a generalised disease. Severe infections and diseases producing dehydration will produce a red eye. In these cases, the underlying cause must also be treated.

Foreign Bodies

Foreign bodies are not very common but, when they do occur, they produce severe irritation and conjunctivitis. Usually only one eye is affected so any dog presented to the vet with severe conjunctivitis of one eye will be closely examined for evidence of foreign material. Grass seeds, for instance, will occasionally lodge behind the nictitating membrane.

Treatment This foreign material must be removed as soon as possible, either under a local or general anaesthetic, and the accompanying conjunctivitis and corneal damage also treated.

Trauma

A severe knock to the eye will often rupture the small blood vessels in the conjunctiva or sclera and produce a haemorrhage which can clearly be seen against the white part of the eye.

Treatment No treatment is necessary provided there is no other damage, but the eye must be kept clean by gentle bathing with warm, sterile saline. The blood clot will be removed quickly by the dog's own defence mechanisms.

DISEASES OF THE CORNEA

Keratitis

Inflammation of the cornea is known as keratitis. In the early stages the cornea appears blue due to the oedema. As the cornea contains no blood vessels at all, these must grow on to the cornea from the edge of the eye to allow healing. This may lead to the eye becoming pigmented and, in severe cases, the dog may become blind. Keratitis is often associated with conjunctivitis, and the most common causes are infection, trauma or any condition which leads to drying of the eye.

Treatment The affected eye is cleaned with cotton wool dipped in sterile water or saline and instilling drops or ointments containing antibiotics and/or anti-inflammatory drugs as directed by the vet.

Pannus

Pannus, which is a type of keratitis of auto-immune origin, is the invasion of the surface

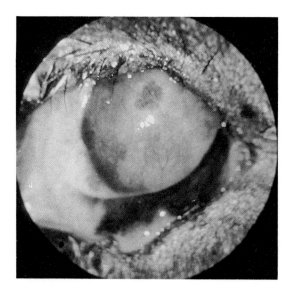

Long-standing keratitis of this right eye.

of the cornea by blood vessels from the outer margin and these appear as a fleshy growth. It seems to occur most commonly in the German Shepherd Dog.

Treatment Anti-inflammatory drops are usually successful but the condition will often recur.

Blue Eye

This is a term used to describe a bluish grey opacity of the cornea, seen following infection with canine infectious hepatitis, or sometimes following injection with a live vaccine. Blue eye usually affects one eye and there is complete loss of vision. Blue eye normally disappears in a few days without treatment but, in severe cases, anti-inflammatory eye drops may prove beneficial.

Corneal Ulcer

An ulcer is an erosion of part of the surface of the cornea and is seen commonly in dogs. Where a corneal ulcer is present, it should be treated as a potentially serious problem as

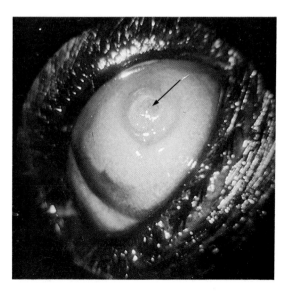

A deep ulcer in the cornea.

it may deepen and rupture the eye. Ulcers are usually caused by scratches to the eye so the short-nosed breeds, such as Pekingese and Shih Tzu, are more susceptible because of their large, unprotected eyes. However, excessive facial folds, for example in the Bulldog and Pekingese, or entropion can also cause ulcers as these conditions involve facial hair rubbing on the cornea.

Corneal ulcers are very painful, and where present, the eyelids are at least partially closed as the eye becomes very inflamed. Some ulcers are quite apparent on close examination but others can only be demonstrated by staining the eye with greenish yellow fluorescein drops which outline the irregular surface of the ulcer.

Treatment Small ulcers can be treated by cleansing the eye with warm, sterile water and instilling antibiotic drops or ointment. Anti-inflammatory drugs are not to be used as they will aggravate the condition. More severe ulcers, or non-healing ulcers, may require cauterisation under a local or general anaesthetic. Following this, the surface of the eye may have to be protected by suturing the nictitating membrane or a flap of conjunctiva across the eye for two weeks in an operation called a keratoplasty.

Most ulcers will heal with treatment but some will leave a faint, grey scar on the cornea. Healing can take a long time with complicated ulcers, in our experience especially in Boxers.

Corneal Dystrophy

This is the presence of a small, faint white shadow in the cornea of one or both eyes. It is caused by a small deposit of fats in the cornea and is usually of no consequence to the dog. It is not normally progressive and causes no loss of sight. In our experience, it seems to occur in Shelties and Rough Collies more often than in other breeds.

Kerato-Conjunctivitis Sicca (Dry Eye)

This is a disease seen principally in the West Highland White Terrier, which develops because of a failure to produce tears. As the cornea dries, keratitis and conjunctivitis develop, and the surface of the eye becomes covered with a grey, sticky mucus. In long-standing cases, the cornea becomes invaded by blood vessels which lead to pigmentation and loss of sight. The condition can occur in one or both eyes. There are several causes, most are auto-immune.

Treatment Artificial tears and anti-inflammatory drops will often control but not cure the condition. As saliva is very similar to tears in composition, it is possible to transplant the parotid duct (a duct carrying saliva from the parotid salivary gland to the mouth) so that it discharges just inside the lower eyelid instead of the mouth. The only problem with this operation is that at feeding time there can be an outpouring of 'tears' causing a very wet face. The dog has an over-abundant supply of salivary glands so this diversion of one of them causes no interference with eating.

Foreign Bodies

Occasionally a fleck of dirt or paint will adhere to the cornea or a thorn may become embedded. If the eye is left untreated, keratitis, and even ulceration, will develop.

Treatment Gentle bathing using sterile warm water may flush the foreign body away but if not it must be removed under a local or general anaesthetic, and post-operative antibiotic cover may be needed.

Dermoids

Dermoids are pink hairy lumps that develop on part of the surface of the cornea, conjunctiva or eyelids. They are congenital, being present at birth, and if they are small they look unsightly but may cause no clinical signs. Large dermoids cause irritation and will impair vision.

Treatment This consists of surgical removal, under a general anaesthetic. The procedure is a very delicate one but the results are usually excellent.

DISEASES OF THE INTERIOR OF THE EYE

Discharges into the anterior chamber can be seen through the cornea as either grey or yellow (caused by pus) or red areas (caused by haemorrhage).

Infection

Occasionally infection will gain entry into the eye from a penetrating wound of the cornea, or a ruptured ulcer. The affected eye fills with pus causing the anterior chamber to appear whitish grey or yellow. The conjunctiva becomes very inflamed, and the eye is painful and almost certainly blind.

Treatment Antibiotics are necessary in an attempt to save the eye, but although the eye is resilient, sight cannot always be restored. If the eye remains blind *and* painful it may be necessary to remove it surgically.

Haemorrhage

A sharp blow to the eye can result in internal bleeding which fills the anterior chamber with blood. At this stage, the eye will be blind but, surprisingly, it may not be particularly painful.

Treatment This involves rest, with antibiotic and anti-inflammatory treatment to prevent infection. In many cases, the blood clot will be slowly reabsorbed leaving little or no damage to the eye.

Uveitis

This is the inflammation of the iris and associated structures and is usually very painful. The eye is inflamed, the lids partially or fully closed and a profuse watery discharge is seen due to excessive tear production. The pupil is small and reacts poorly to light, the iris appears dull and pus may be present in the anterior chamber. The cause of uveitis is not always obvious, but can result from infection or an immune reaction.

Treatment   Uveitis is treated with anti-inflammatory drugs and it may be necessary to use them both locally onto the surface of the eye and as injections or tablets. In addition, drops which dilate the pupil are used to prevent the iris from adhering to the lens. Severe uveitis may so damage the eye that glaucoma develops because the drainage of the eye becomes impaired.

Glaucoma

Glaucoma results when an increase in the fluid pressure of the aqueous occurs inside the eye and is often sudden in onset. In the early stages the only sign may be a slightly inflamed eye with a little discharge, but the affected eye may appear enlarged or prominent. As the pressure increases, the condition becomes more painful and the eyelids may be partially closed. The eye appears very inflamed, excessive tear production occurs and the dilated pupil shows no light reflex. The cornea becomes opaque and later is invaded by blood vessels. If untreated, the eye becomes grossly enlarged and eyesight fails. There are two types of glaucoma:

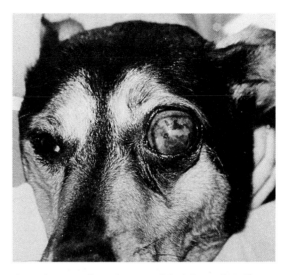

Severe long-standing glaucoma of the left eye of a Jack Russell Terrier.

Primary glaucoma   In certain breeds, such as the Basset Hound, Springer and English Cocker Spaniel, glaucoma can develop with no underlying disease.

Secondary glaucoma   This type of glaucoma follows another primary problem such as lens luxation or uveitis.

Glaucoma is diagnosed on clinical signs and by measurement of the internal pressure of the eye (tonometry).

Treatment   This is never easy. The most effective initial treatment is the use of drugs in an attempt to reduce the production of aqueous. In many cases surgery is required to establish drainage of the eye. The operation consists of trephining (drilling) a small hole through the sclera beneath the conjunctiva. Treatment is not always successful and where the eye has become blind, it may be necessary to remove it surgically to eliminate the pain.

Tumours

Tumours inside the eye are very uncommon and, when they occur, they usually affect only one eye. Lymphosarcoma tumours, however, can affect both eyes. The pupil will become grey and dull, vision will deteriorate, and as the tumour progresses, the eye may become inflamed and painful.

Treatment Surgical removal of the affected eyeball is usually successful if performed in the early stages before the tumour has spread to other tissues surrounding the eye.

DISEASES OF THE LENS

Cataract

A cataract is an opacity of the lens and may occur in one or, more usually, both eyes. The pupil appears whitish instead of the normal black colour, and in advanced cases the lens looks like a pearl. The process of cataract formation is normally very slow and the degree of lens opacity will determine the effect on vision. Many dogs with some cataract formation lead perfectly normal lives, whereas others are completely blind. A senile change in the lens of the older dog, called nuclear sclerosis, can resemble cataract but does not cause loss of vision.

There are many causes of cataract and these include infection, diabetes mellitus, trauma and inherited causes. Breeds which suffer from inherited cataract include the Golden Retriever, Labrador, Boston Terrier, American Cocker Spaniel and Afghan Hound. The dogs are not born with the disease but the cataract develops in the young adult. A British Veterinary Association/Kennel Club (BVA/KC) Eye Scheme exists to detect early cataracts in breeding dogs in order to prevent further

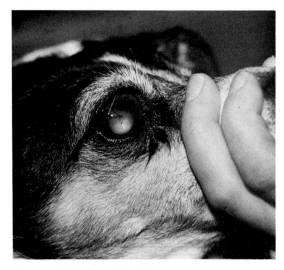

A cataract in the lens of the right eye.

spread by using affected animals. All dogs belonging to breeds known to have a high risk of inherited eye disease should be examined on this scheme before breeding is considered.

Treatment Once a cataract has developed the only treatment is surgical removal. However, this is only recommended for dogs with severely impaired vision caused by mature cataracts in both eyes.

As cataract may accompany other causes of blindness such as retinal atrophy, it is essential to ensure that the eye is otherwise normal before considering surgery. Only one cataract is removed usually as this gives adequate vision.

Lens Luxation

This is seen occasionally in certain breeds, especially the Tibetan Terrier, Fox Terrier, Jack Russell Terrier and Sealyham. The ligament suspending the lens breaks because of an inherited weakness, and the lens can fall either into the anterior or posterior chamber. Lens luxation can also be caused by a severe blow to the eye.

A prolapsed lens in the posterior chamber will often cause little damage and may be difficult to diagnose. There may be some loss of sight and a dilated pupil. Removal from this site is extremely difficult and usually not necessary.

A forward displacement of the lens into the anterior chamber will very quickly produce glaucoma with all the associated signs (*see* page 139).

Treatment   If the lens has displaced into the anterior chamber it must be removed surgically as soon as possible to save the sight. If neglected, the sight will certainly be lost and the eye itself may have to be removed surgically if glaucoma develops.

DISEASES OF THE RETINA

Diseases of the retina may seriously impair vision and are, unfortunately, common in the dog.

Progressive Retinal Atrophy (PRA)

PRA is a term used to describe a number of inherited progressive degenerations of the light-sensitive layer of the eye which may lead to total blindness. In the early stages, the pupil dilates in an attempt to let more light into the eye as the vision becomes defective. The condition, which is painless, is diagnosed by a veterinary examination of the back of the eye with an ophthalmoscope. There are two types of PRA:

Generalised PRA   Degeneration initially leads to the loss of peripheral vision and night blindness but progresses to total blindness. It is seen in breeds such as the Cocker Spaniel, Irish Setter and Miniature and Toy Poodles. It is caused by a recessive gene and therefore only occurs in puppies whose parents are both carriers.

Central PRA   Pigmented areas develop throughout the retina causing a loss of detailed vision but this condition rarely develops to complete blindness. The dog can see moving objects but may miss still ones. Central PRA is seen mainly in the Briard, Labrador, Golden Retriever, Border Collie and Rough and Smooth Collies.

Prevention   There is no treatment for PRA and the disease must be controlled by the testing of breeding stock. Affected individuals must not be used for breeding.

Collie Eye Anomaly

This is a disease of the Rough and Smooth Collies and Sheltie in which there are various defects present in the eye at birth which can be seen with an ophthalmoscope. In many cases, there may be no noticeable loss of vision, but partial or total blindness can occur as the result of retinal detachment.

Prevention   There is no treatment and the disease must be controlled by the testing of breeding stock. Affected dogs should not be used for breeding.

Retinal Detachment

The retina separates from the back of the eye and causes complete and sudden blindness, usually in only one eye. It can be caused by a knock but often occurs as a sequel to another problem such as inflammation, a prolapsed lens, or PRA. There is currently no treatment available once the retina has detached.

12 The Locomotor System

The locomotor system comprises the bones, joints, ligaments, tendons and muscles. Its function is to support, protect and move the body.

NORMAL STRUCTURE AND FUNCTION

The bones form the hard framework of the body to which the ligaments, muscles and tendons are attached. There are 319 separate bones in the dog. A typical long bone, such as the femur, consists of a middle portion, the shaft, and two ends, the epiphyses. The shaft consists of an outer hard layer of calcified tissue called the cortex and a central cavity, the marrow cavity, which is filled with marrow. In some bones this contributes to the production of blood cells. The ends of the bone, or epiphyses, have a thinner outer layer which is filled with a supporting

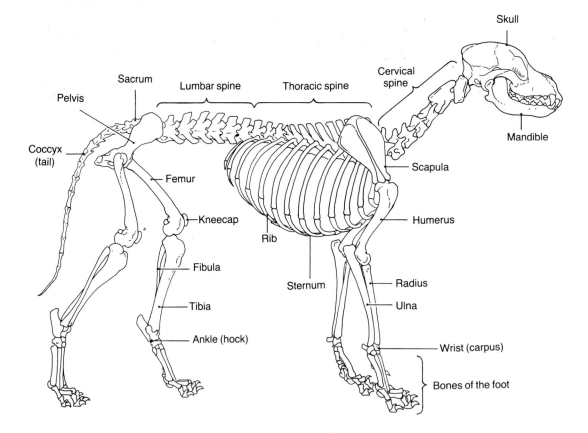

Fig 28 Skeleton of a dog

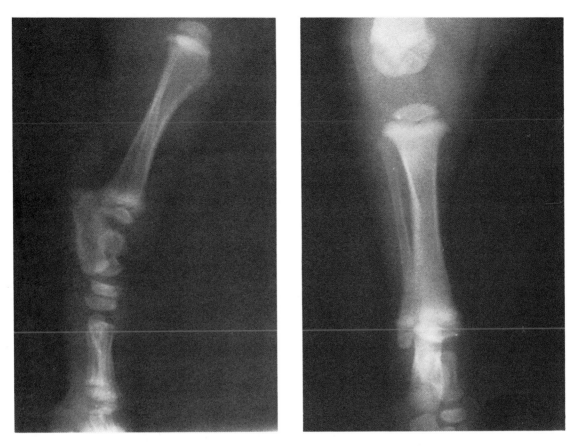

Young bone showing wide joints composed mainly of cartilage. The growth plates are clearly visible.

framework of softer cancellous, or porous bone.

Bone is produced by the calcification of a cartilage template, a process called ossification, and for this an adequate supply of calcium, phosphorus and vitamin D is essential. Flat bones and small bones develop from a single centre of ossification but long bones grow from either end at a special cartilage layer, called the growth plate, which separates the shaft from the epiphysis. Bone is a living tissue and, once formed, is still capable of slowly changing shape in response to stresses and strains that are put upon it.

A joint is formed where two or more bones meet and articulate with one another. At the joint, the ends of the bones are covered by shiny, smooth cartilage which allows them to slide over each other without damage. This cartilage is enclosed by a joint capsule which produces a viscous fluid, called synovial fluid, to oil the joint. Ligaments are strands of fibrous tissue which link bones together at joints and hold them in place.

Muscles consist of masses of small contractile filaments which, when they all contract together, shorten the muscle. At any time, even in a resting muscle, a few fibres are contracting and this gives a muscle 'tone'. Each muscle has its own blood and nerve supply and is attached at each end to bone either directly or by fibrous tissue, called tendons. Tendons can vary in shape – some are flat and wide while others are round –

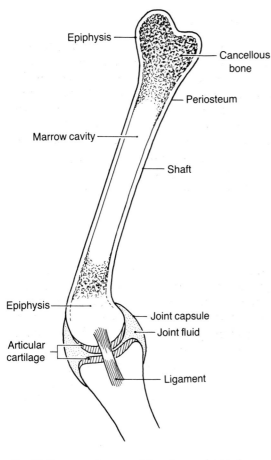

Fig 29 Structure of a normal long bone and typical joint

and they can be long or short. The longest tendons are those moving the toes. Muscles can have other functions as well as locomotion. For example, the intercostal muscles between the ribs, and the diaphragm muscle enable the dog to breathe, while contraction of the abdominal muscles helps in defaecation, urination and birth.

LAMENESS

Lameness is an important clinical sign in the diagnosis of locomotor disorders. A study of the type and severity of lameness is of great help to the vet in reaching a diagnosis. Some conditions can be diagnosed almost by watching the dog walk.

Lameness can be sudden in onset or it may develop gradually over a long period. It may be so mild that it is difficult to detect which leg is lame or it may affect a leg so severely that the dog cannot put it to the ground. Lameness may affect a single leg, two legs or more.

Fractures, dislocations or sprains are normally sudden in onset and usually affect a single leg. However, if lameness develops in a leg over a period of time, the vet will normally look for another cause, such as a developmental abnormality, a bone tumour or arthritis resulting from an accident. If more than one leg is affected, especially in the older dog, degenerative arthritis may be suspected.

Most lamenesses are associated with pain and the site of the pain indicates to the vet the location of the injury. Occasionally, however, a dog may be severely lame but show no pain reflex at all. An example of this would be a dog with a ruptured cruciate ligament in the stifle or knee joint.

Some abnormalities of balance may resemble lameness, such as ataxia where the dog walks as if he is drunk. This is caused by damage to the nervous system, possibly due to poisoning or damage to the inner ear or brain itself.

Lameness, of course, is not always due to damage to the locomotor system. A thorn in the pad or an inter-digital abscess can cause a very acute lameness and therefore a detailed examination of an affected leg may be necessary. If the dog is very tense or suffering great pain, sedation or even a general anaesthetic may be required for this examination.

DISEASES OF BONE

Metabolic Disease

This type of bone disorder is seen almost exclusively in the young growing dog. Therefore, the next five problems are discussed in greater detail in Chapter 4.

Juvenile Osteoporosis

This is a disease of puppies caused by a lack of calcium or an excess of phosphorus in the diet which results in the formation of weak bones. (*See* Chapter 4, page 48).

Rickets

Rickets is caused by a diet lacking in calcium, phosphorus and vitamin D. There is damage to the growth plate which results in swelling of the bone ends, weak joints and bowing of the legs. It is very uncommon. (*See* Chapter 4, page 48.)

Hypertrophic Osteodystrophy

This is an uncommon but painful disease which occurs in the larger breeds of dog between four and eight months of age. It affects the growing ends of bones, causing the joints to swell and become hot and painful. The dog may be left with enlarged joints, especially those at the lower end of the limbs. (*See* Chapter 4, page 49.)

Femoral Head Necrosis

This is a disease of unknown cause, affecting the growth of one or both hip joints in small breeds, especially the Jack Russell Terrier. There is a degeneration of the bone of the head of the femur producing severe pain and collapse of the joint. In some cases, damage to the blood supply to this small piece of bone is thought to be the cause. (*See* Chapter 4, page 52.)

Failure of Bones to Fuse

Some of the larger bones have bony projections which develop from smaller centres of ossification and then fuse with the main bone when maturity is reached. Two common problems are seen in the larger breeds, both occurring in the elbow joint. These are ununited anconeal process and ununited coronoid process, both of which produce a gradually developing, painful lameness in the foreleg. (*See* Chapter 4, pages 50 and 51.)

Rubber Jaw

This is a condition where the bones become soft due to excessive mineral loss in chronic kidney failure (*see also* Chapter 14, page 176). The disease is most readily noticed in the softening of the lower jaw bone, hence the name. There is no specific treatment for this as the problem is primarily due to kidney failure which may, or may not, respond to treatment. It is usually a disease of the older dog.

Craniomandibular Osteoarthropathy or Lion-Head Disease

This is an uncommon disease seen almost invariably in the young, growing West Highland White Terrier or Scottish Terrier and it is characterised by symmetrical bony enlargements on the dorsal skull and mandible. The disease is painful initially and the puppy, who may be reluctant to eat, salivates and has a raised temperature.

Treatment The disease is self-limiting and at maturity, at about nine months of age, no more new bone is produced. The dog is then left with painless, bony masses on the skull and jaw. During the active phase the pain can be controlled with pain-killing drugs.

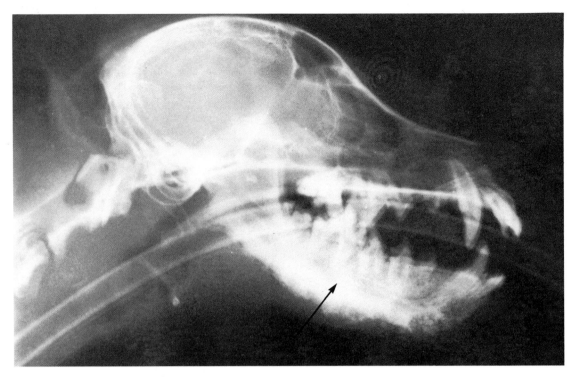

An X-ray of a West Highland White Terrier with craniomandibular osteoarthropathy. The lower jaw is severely affected.

Atrophy

If a bone is not subjected to its normal stresses, for example because of a chronic lameness, it will become partially demineralised and therefore weaker. This is called atrophy and on an X-ray the bone will look greyer. This atrophy will slow down the healing of any accompanying fracture.

Bone Cysts

Bone cysts are uncommon but they are seen in the long bones, especially the radius of puppies of the larger breeds. The puppy will be lame and there will be a swelling on the leg over the cyst. The cyst will weaken the bone which may fracture at this site.

Treatment The cyst can be treated by removing it surgically from the bone. The leg is then supported by, for instance, a splint while the cavity fills with new bone.

Infections

Bone infection (osteomyelitis) is caused when bacteria invade the bone, usually as a sequel to trauma such as a bite, or the protrusion of the end of a broken bone through the skin. In the toe, infection can invade the bone by gaining access through a damaged nail bed. Occasionally, osteomyelitis can occur as a primary infection with no obvious cause. Bone infections are normally localised to one part of a single bone.

Usually the first indication of osteomyelitis is pain, accompanied by heat and swelling over the site of the infection in the bone. If a limb bone is affected, there can be severe lameness. As the disease progresses the dog will become lethargic, off his food and may have a raised temperature. Sometimes, the infection will extend outwards to the skin to produce a discharging wound. Extensive osteomyelitis may weaken the bone to such a point that it may fracture.

Diagnosis Radiography is necessary to reach a diagnosis and osteomyelitis will show as an irregular erosion in the bone. This is diagnostic when accompanied by the above symptoms.

Treatment Large doses of the appropriate antibiotic for several weeks are essential but, occasionally, it will be necessary to remove the diseased portion of bone surgically. Severe osteomyelitis of the small bones of a toe, arising from a nail-bed infection, may require amputation of the toe.

To prevent osteomyelitis following a deep wound or compound fracture, immediate and thorough cleansing of the site is necessary with adequate antibiotic cover.

Fractures

Any break or crack in a bone is called a fracture. There are six types:

Fissure fracture The bone is only cracked and there is no displacement at the fracture site.
Greenstick fracture The break in the bone is incomplete. The bone may bend but part of the fractured bone remains intact, exactly as a green, new branch of a tree would break.
Simple fracture The bone is completely broken at one site into two separate pieces.
Comminuted fracture The bone is broken into several pieces.
Compound fracture A broken end of bone penetrates the skin.
Folding fracture The bone is so weak that it just collapses or bends.

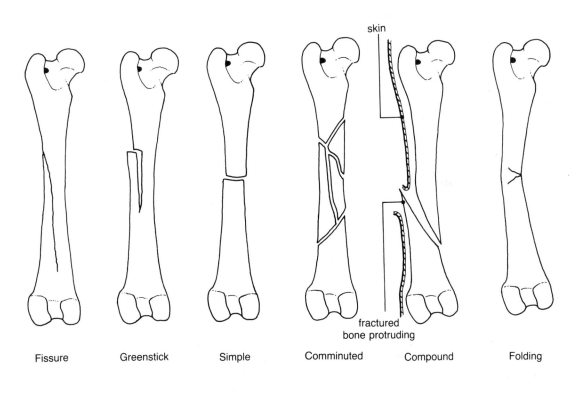

Fissure Greenstick Simple Comminuted Compound Folding

Fig 30 Types of fracture

The larger bones require a substantial force to break them and broken bones are usually the result of accidents. The most common causes are road traffic accidents, puppies being accidentally trodden on and small dogs being dropped. Bones most commonly involved are the femur, pelvis, radius and ulna, tibia and fibula and bones of the feet. The bones of the skull surrounding the brain are very rarely fractured in dogs. Bones which have become weakened by disease such as cysts, tumours, infection or by a poor diet may fracture with very little force or they may just simply fold to produce a bent limb.

Pain is a feature of all fractures and even a minor fracture will cause the animal to be lame. In addition, both heat and swelling are usually present over the fracture site. If the bone is completely broken, the leg below the fracture will be floppy and bone may be seen protruding through the skin. Sometimes fractures may cause severe injury to other organs as in the case of a rib puncturing a lung or a fractured vertebra compressing the spinal cord to produce paralysis. The jagged end of a fractured leg bone may sever nerves or blood vessels.

Diagnosis This is usually straightforward as the vet, presented with a lame dog with a history of an accident, may be able to palpate the fracture. Some fractures, however, are more difficult to diagnose, especially fissure or greenstick fractures in very small puppies. As puppies will rarely keep still during a clinical examination, especially if in pain, sedation or anaesthesia may be necessary. If a fracture is suspected, radiography will confirm this and locate the site.

Except for compound fractures with the danger of infection, it is not necessary to perform surgery to repair fractures immediately. Other more serious problems such as shock, haemorrhage or damage to internal organs which are more life threatening must be treated first. Only when the dog is in a stable condition will an anaesthetic be administered and the fracture repaired. However, a temporary splint may be used to support the fractured leg and keep the dog comfortable until surgery is possible. Where certain bones such as the pelvis are fractured, confinement in a hospital kennel gives relief from discomfort.

Treatment When a vet repairs a fracture, his aim is to place the fractured ends of bone into their normal position and then immobilise the bone for approximately six weeks. Methods available are cage rest, external casts or surgery to perform internal fixation.

1 **Cage rest** This is suitable for fractured bones which have little displacement and are well supported by muscle. Many pelvic fractures can be treated in this way.

2 **External support** External support is only really suitable for fractures of the lower legs, such as those involving the radius/ulna, tibia/fibula and fractures of the feet. Various types of external support are available but to be effective, the support must 'fit' closely to the limb without being too tight and it must immobilise the joints above and below the fracture. Plaster of Paris, which is applied wet but dries to form a solid support is perhaps the most frequently used cast but this type has its drawbacks. A dog may chew through it, it may get wet and crumble, or because the dog may be too active or the leg may swell, rub or pressure sores may develop under it. Alternatives available to the vet include padded splints, and newer plastic materials which can be moulded while soft to fit the leg. The support is normally applied for a minimum of four weeks, ideally six, but sometimes it may be necessary to replace it periodically. This applies particularly to growing puppies or compound fractures. We prefer to check patients with external casts on a weekly basis.

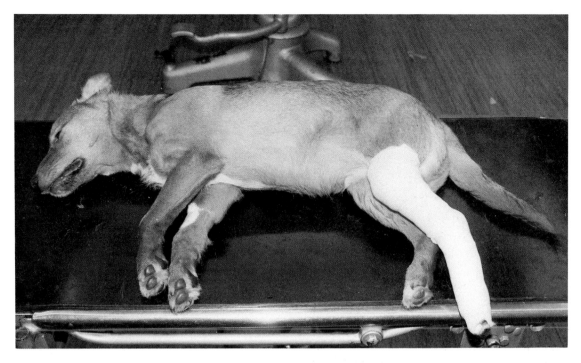

An external support has been applied to this dog with a fracture of the lower end of his tibia.

3 **Internal fixation** Fractures which cannot be stabilised with external casts will require surgery to fix the broken fragments in close apposition. The most common methods of internal fixation are intramedullary pins, bone plates and screws, small pins and wire, and single screws.

Intramedullary pins can be used in the larger straight bones such as the femur and humerus. The pin is inserted into one of the broken ends and then pushed out through the top of the bone. The fracture is then reduced and the pin pushed into the other portion of bone to hold it in place. Any excess pin is removed where it protrudes from the top of the bone.

In more complicated fractures, or if the bone is one without a marrow cavity, the vet may prefer to use a bone plate and screws. The plate is applied on the outside of the bone and is fixed to either side of the fracture by screws. The holes are drilled in the bone using a sterile drill.

Small, displaced fragments of bone can be re-attached using small stainless steel pins, stainless steel wire or single screws. Such fractures usually occur near the ends of bones.

In most fractures, the pin or plate is left in place even after the fracture has healed. Occasionally a dog will reject the metal, which may need to be removed. This procedure is not always straightforward.

Most fractures will be fully healed after about six weeks and if the immobilised bones have not been disturbed, the dog will normally become perfectly fit again. However, despite correct immobilisation some fractures fail to heal. This may be due to infection, or because the fractured ends are non-viable as a result of the accident. In toy breeds, especially the Toy Poodle, it is well recognised that fractures of the lower radius/ulna are very slow to heal. If the fracture fails to heal, a painful false joint develops at

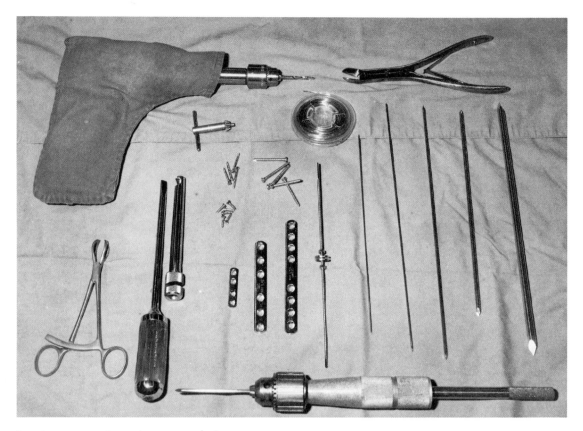

Bone instruments, plates, pins, screws and wire.

the fracture site resulting in abnormal movement. To stabilise these false joints, it is necessary to perform surgery to remove the section of non-healing bone and then fix the bone ends together with a bone plate and screws. In very rare cases, fractures will never heal and it may be necessary to amputate the leg.

Folding fractures are impossible to treat with complete success at the time of injury, due to the weakness of the bone. Correction of the diet is of paramount importance to strengthen and re-mineralise the bones and cage rest is essential to prevent further fractures. Such patients are usually left with deformed limbs.

Damage to the Growth Plate

The growth plate in young growing puppies is an area of weakness and can be easily damaged. In some cases, damage to the growth plate will cause growth at that end of the bone to cease so that limb will then be shorter than its opposite number. However, if two bones are growing alongside each other and one bone stops growing while the other bone continues normally, the leg will bend as it grows. This is a particular problem of the lower end of the radius/ulna of large dogs, such as Great Danes and Irish Wolfhounds, from about five months of age. It will produce a marked deviation of the foreleg at the wrist called Carpus valgus.

Sometimes, a fracture will occur precisely through a growth plate. In our experience,

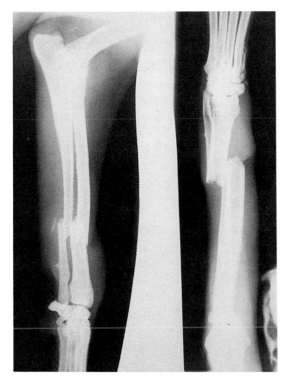

Two X-ray views of a fractured radius and ulna.

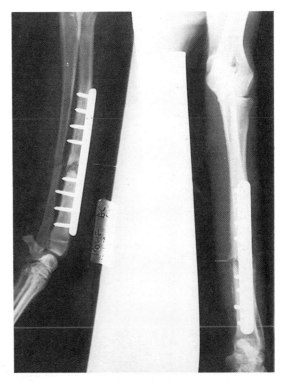

The same fractures repaired with a bone plate and screws.

this occurs most commonly at the lower end of the femur and is called a supracondylar fracture. The fractured end must be reattached surgically for normal growth to continue in the affected puppy.

Bone Tumours

Bone tumours are not very common, except in the giant breeds such as the Great Dane and Irish Wolfhound, where they tend to occur at certain sites. The most common sites are in the radius above the wrist joint, in the humerus below the shoulder and in the femur above the stifle. Initially, the only symptom is a slight limp and the dog may become very lame before any swelling develops at the tumour site.

Diagnosis X-ray examination or biopsy will reveal the typical erosive nature of the tumour. Bone tumours are extremely painful

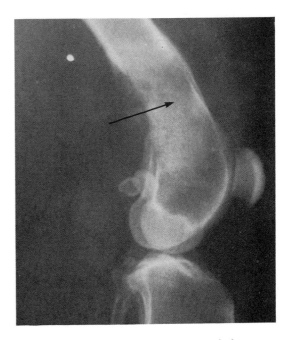

An osteosarcoma bone tumour of the lower end of the femur.

and this pain is very difficult to control with the drugs normally used in lameness cases. The tumours tend to be highly malignant and spread to other parts of the body early in the course of the disease.

Treatment Amputation of the limb will remove the primary tumour and give temporary relief of pain but as the tumour may have already spread to other areas, it is not normally recommended. Other forms of treatment such as radiotherapy and chemotherapy are not normally successful, but in certain types of tumour may be worth trying.

DISEASES OF JOINTS

Sprains

A sprain is an inflammation of a joint and is caused when the joint is over-stretched, for example by an awkward fall. A mild sprain results in a hot, swollen, painful joint and some degree of lameness.

Treatment This is treated with rest, cold compresses and perhaps mild pain-killing drugs, such as Paracetamol. The symptoms usually disappear within a few days.

A more severe sprain may result in tearing of the joint capsule or ligaments causing more severe swelling and lameness. Even severe sprains will usually heal with rest but a supporting bandage and anti-inflammatory drugs may be necessary to reduce the pain and speed the healing process.

Severe trauma to a joint may rupture the ligaments and produce an unstable, painful joint. The dog will be very lame on that leg and may unable to place any weight on it at all.

Treatment In most cases surgical repair will be necessary.

Ruptured Cruciate Ligament

The anterior and posterior cruciate ligaments are present in the stifle or knee joint and as this is a very shallow joint, their function is to prevent the bones of the stifle joint from moving forwards and backwards in relation to each other. When they rupture as a result of a severe sprain, the joint is destabilised and the dog becomes totally lame on that leg. This occurs most commonly in middle-aged overweight dogs whose excess weight gives added momentum to a sprain and ruptures the ligament. At the time of the injury, the dog is often trying to jump and turn at the same time but he suddenly cries out in pain and carries the leg. The initial pain and swelling, however, rapidly diminish but the lameness persists.

Diagnosis The injury is diagnosed by

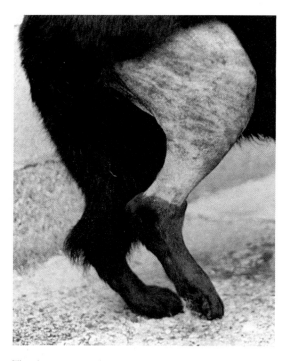

The classic stance of a dog with a ruptured cruciate ligament (the leg has been shaved prior to surgery).

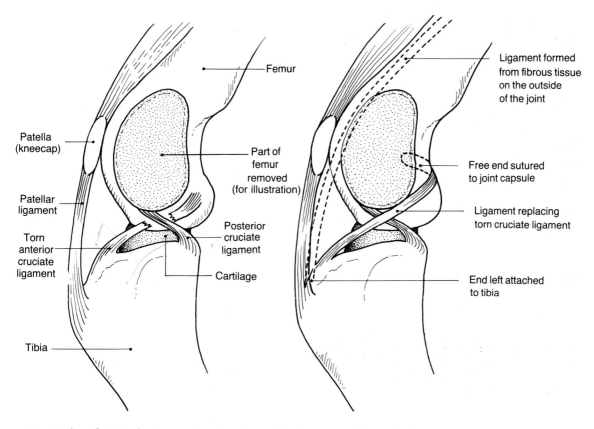

Fig 31 The stifle joint showing a ruptured anterior cruciate ligament and the authors' method of repair

demonstrating the excessive movement of the joint which results from rupture of this ligament, the so-called 'drawer-movement'. To ensure the dog is totally relaxed, it will often be necessary to give an anaesthetic to elicit this movement.

Treatment In the smaller breeds, if strict rest is enforced for about two months, the joint may stabilise and the dog become sound. However, if no improvement is seen after a short time, it will be necessary to replace the ligament surgically. In medium to large breeds, surgical repair is usually necessary and a variety of techniques involving natural and artificial ligaments are available to your vet. The results are usually very good. The post-operative recovery is slow and the patient must be kept very quiet, especially for the first few weeks after the operation. If the joint is not repaired and remains unstable, it will become severely arthritic, and the dog very lame.

Dislocations (Luxations)

Dislocations occur when there is total rupture of the ligaments and joint capsule of a joint allowing the bones to separate. The cause is a severe blow or twist, usually sustained in a road accident. In our experience, the joint most commonly dislocated is the hip, followed by the elbow, shoulder

153

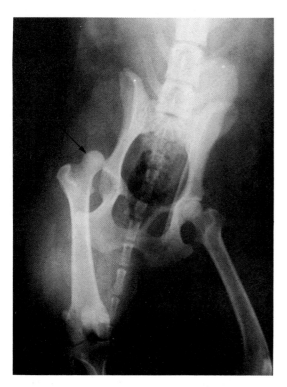

An X-ray showing the dog has a dislocated right hip.

and, to a much lesser extent, the hock joint. Dislocation of the patella or kneecap is an example of a partial dislocation of a joint. The femur and tibia usually remain in place while the patella moves out of its groove to the inside aspect of the leg. Dislocations are characterised by severe pain and sudden lameness following trauma.

Treatment The luxated bone must be replaced as soon as possible after the injury, before tissue swelling, haemorrhage and muscle contraction make the reduction more difficult or impossible. Reduction of a dislocated joint is usually carried out under a general anaesthetic, and afterwards the joint may need support for several days. Sometimes, the damage to the tissues around the joint is so severe that it repeatedly re-dislocates after replacement.

In cases such as this involving the hip joint, surgery is necessary in order to stabilise the joint using a technique known as toggling.

Infection (Septic Arthritis)

Joint infections are rare in dogs and when they occur, they are usually caused by penetrating wounds. The clinical signs are severe pain, heat and swelling of a joint, a wound is invariably present and the dog is lame. Usually, only one joint is involved. In severe cases, the dog will be lethargic and off his food.

Diagnosis An X-ray will show the charact-eristic changes, and the withdrawal of a small sample of joint fluid by the vet for laboratory testing will confirm the diagnosis. In severe infections, the damage to the joint will result in a chronic arthritis.

Treatment Antibiotic sensitivity testing of the joint fluid will identify the drug to use and this will normally be used in high doses for a prolonged course.

Osteoarthritis

In this book we are using the term osteo-arthritis to mean a chronic degeneration of a joint, which results in thickening of the capsule, formation of new bone around the edges of the joint and, sometimes, erosion of the joint cartilage. An arthritic joint is initially enlarged and painful and it has a reduced range of movement. Arthritis can result from earlier damage to a joint, such as infection, a sprain, or cruciate ligament damage but it can also occur as a result of deformed joints, as for example in hip dysplasia.

Osteoarthritis tends to be a disease of the older, larger dog and is most commonly a problem of the hips, stifles and elbows. If arthritis is present in a single joint, the dog will be lame on that leg, the degree of

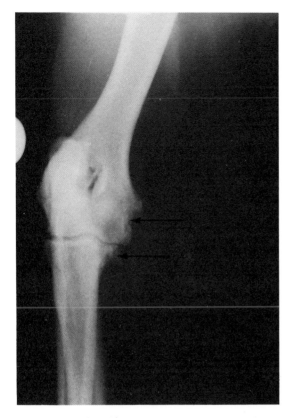

Osteoarthritis of the elbow joint.

lameness reflecting the severity of the arthritis. If more than one joint is affected, the dog will have difficulty in rising and sitting and he will be generally slow. As the arthritis progresses, the dog will spend more time lying down until he may become completely recumbent, or only able to stand with great difficulty. Generally, arthritis is at its worst after the dog has rested. Once he has moved around a little, he seems to be able to move more freely.

Spondylitis can be regarded as arthritis of the spine. This condition is fairly common in the older, larger dog and produces symptoms similar to arthritis of the hip. However, in the Boxer, spondylitis can occur at a young age and can be extremely painful and difficult to treat.

Treatment There is no cure for arthritis once the joint surface is affected and treatment is aimed at alleviating the pain with anti-inflammatory drugs. Arthritic dogs should not be allowed to become overweight and great attention should be paid to diet. They should not be subjected to long walks; several short walks daily are

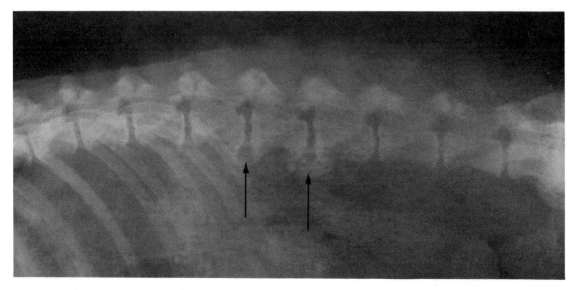

Spondylitis of the spine.

preferable. Undue exposure to cold and wet weather should also be avoided, and old dogs with spondylitis of the spine or severe hip arthritis may need coats in adverse weather.

Prevention It is important to try to eliminate the causes of arthritis as once it has occurred it is impossible to cure. Prompt attention to sprains and joint infections, attention to diet to ensure the dog is not overweight, especially as middle age approaches, and the reduction in the numbers of dogs with hereditary joint abnormalities are all important factors.

Hip Dysplasia (HD)

Hip dysplasia is a very common and serious developmental abnormality of the hip joint affecting most of the larger breeds of dog. It is, however, increasingly being seen in some of the smaller breeds. The cause of hip dysplasia is not completely known. Inherited factors are important but other factors such as over supplementation or, conversely, poor nutrition, over-exercise and being overweight during the growing phase will all contribute. It is uncommon in mongrels.

The hip joint is known as a ball and socket joint and this arrangement permits a wide range of movement. The joint is composed of a deep, cup-shaped socket, the acetabulum, in the pelvis into which fits the rounded end, the femoral head, of the femur. In the normal hip there is a very close fit between the femoral head and the socket. When hip dysplasia is present, there is a shallow acetabulum, a distorted femoral head and a slackness of the joint capsule. This allows excess movement between the two bones which gradually gives rise to an unstable, painful joint. This joint, in addition to functioning incorrectly, will gradually become arthritic.

The severity of the symptoms seen in dogs with hip dysplasia usually reflects the degree of malformation of the joint. Mild cases may show no clinical signs at all until arthritis develops later in life, at about eight years of age. A severely affected puppy, however, may hardly be able to walk or to rise from a sitting position when he is as young as five months. When presented with any large dog that has a poor hind leg gait and shows pain in the hip area, the vet will consider the possibility of hip dysplasia.

Diagnosis This is usually based on the breed, age and clinical symptoms. It is confirmed by X-rays and manipulation of the joint under general anaesthesia. Treatment cannot cure hip dysplasia so our aim must be prevention by examining and X-raying all large pedigree dogs intended for breeding. Potential breeding stock of both sexes should be X-rayed at not less than one year of age. These X-rays should then be submitted for scrutiny via the joint British Veterinary Association/Kennel Club (BVA/KC) hip dysplasia scheme. This scheme was established to reduce the incidence of hip dysplasia by encouraging the breeding of dogs with normal hips. The X-rays, bearing the KC registration number of the dog, are examined by a panel of specialist vets who allocate scores to the various parts of each hip joint depending on its shape and structure. Each hip can be scored from 0 to 54, making a total of 108 maximum for the two hips. The lower the score the better and indeed 0:0 is the best score possible. A dog is acceptable for breeding if he scores a total of 8 or less, with a maximum of 6 in any one hip. If a dog has a higher score he should not be used for breeding except as part of a carefully controlled programme in one of the breeds in which the low scores are hardly ever seen. Anyone purchasing a puppy from a breed known to be highly susceptible to hip dysplasia, such as the Labrador, Retriever or Rottweiler, should ensure both parents have been X-rayed and scored. Although

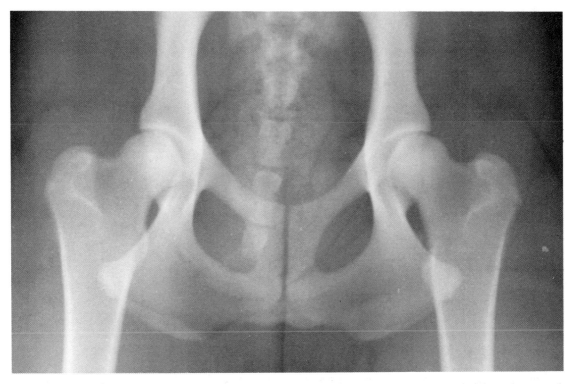

X-ray of a German Shepherd with normal hips. Total score: 0.

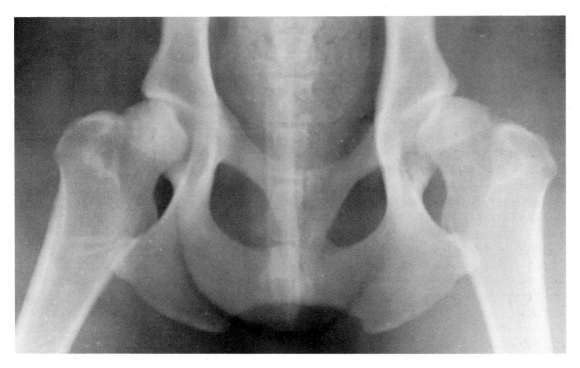

X-ray of a German Shepherd with severe Hip Dysplasia. Total score: 53.

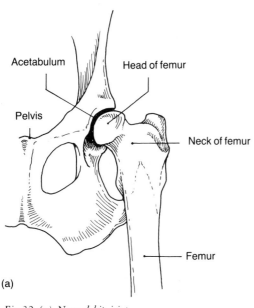

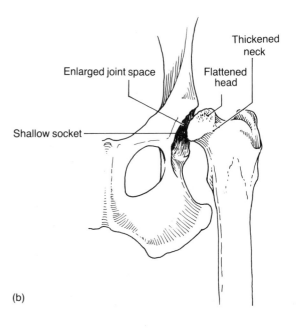

Fig 32 (a) Normal hip joint
(b) Severe hip dysplasia

this is not an absolute guarantee that the puppy will not suffer from hip dysplasia, it will considerably reduce the chances.

Treatment In mild cases of hip dysplasia in puppies, attention to diet and a restricted exercise regime may be sufficient to allow the joint to stabilise. In severe cases in the young dog, surgery will be necessary. Several surgical techniques are available for reducing the pain and improving the lameness. The most common operation performed in general practice is excision arthroplasty. In this operation the femoral head is removed flush with the shaft of the femur. A non-painful false joint develops from fibrous tissue. The recovery period for this operation is about two months. If both hips require surgery, an interval of about three months is left between each operation. Once arthritis has developed, hip dysplasia is then treated as an arthritic problem.

Osteochondritis Dissicans (OCD)

This disease is characterised by degeneration of the cartilage in certain joints of young dogs six to ten months old. It is only seen in the larger breeds of dogs. As the disease affects only adolescent dogs, it is discussed fully in Chapter 4, The Growing Dog (*see* page 51).

Dislocating Patella (Luxating Patella)

This common problem in the toy breeds occurs where a deformity of the stifle joint results in the patella slipping to either side of the joint, instead of remaining centrally in the trochlea groove at the lower end of the femur. This is regarded as an hereditary disease. However, a patella can also dislocate if its supporting ligaments are torn during an accident.

There are a whole range of clinical signs. Some dogs show little or no lameness except

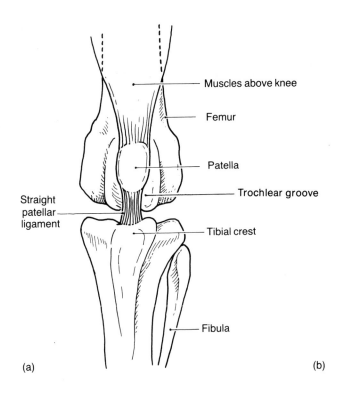

Muscles above knee

Femur

Patella

Trochlear groove

Straight patellar ligament

Tibial crest

Fibula

(a)

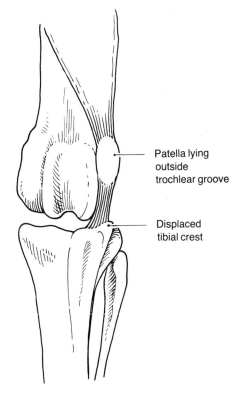

Patella lying outside trochlear groove

Displaced tibial crest

(b)

Fig 33 (a) Normal stifle joint (front view)
(b) Dislocating patella

for a slightly crouching gait. In other cases, the patella slips in and out of position intermittently causing the dog to hold the leg raised for a short time until the patella is replaced. In a severe case, the joint will be painful, have a restricted range of movement and may become arthritic.

In a conscious dog, it is not possible for the vet to push a normal patella out of position, so if this is possible on examining a patient, the joint is abnormal and unstable. An anaesthetic may sometimes be required for this diagnostic test but in most cases of congenital patella luxation, this procedure is painless.

Treatment If a dog's patella luxates intermittently, the owner can perform simple first aid to replace it. The leg should be

straightened gently by holding the foot in one hand and pushing the knee backwards with the other hand. As the leg straightens, the patella will slip back into place. This procedure is not painful to the dog. Surgical correction is necessary in recurrent or painful cases and several techniques are available, depending on the severity of the condition. Mild cases respond well to surgery to shorten the stretched ligament on the opposite side of the joint to which the patella dislocates. More serious or frequent dislocations indicate that the trochlea groove on the femur may be too shallow and require surgery to deepen it. In very severely affected dogs where hereditary factors have caused malformation of the stifle, an operation known as tibial crest transplant will be necessary to realign the point of attachment

159

of the patella. During the development of such a joint, the tibial crest migrates to an abnormal position on the tibia and, as the patella ligaments are attached to this, they pull the patella out of place when the joint flexes.

DISEASES OF MUSCLES AND TENDONS

Strains

A strain is a tear in either a muscle or a tendon and it is usually caused by over-exertion. A strained muscle is swollen, hot and painful and there is some degree of lameness. Most dogs with mild strains will recover with rest alone, but the treatment of more severe strains may also involve the use of anti-inflammatory drugs. Dogs very rarely tear muscles severely enough to require surgery.

Trauma

Muscles and tendons, especially those of the lower legs and feet, are frequently damaged by trauma such as road accidents, cuts and bites. The resulting degree of lameness depends on the muscle affected and the depth of the injury. However, even very shallow wounds in the feet may completely sever the small tendons to the toes resulting in loss of function of one or more toes unless the severed ends are located and repaired immediately. The most severe tendon injury we see is the complete rupture of the Achilles tendon of the hock. This results in the sudden, complete loss of function of that leg and the whole of the lower part of the leg from the hock will lie flat on the ground. This injury is usually caused by the Achilles tendon pulling away from the bone in the hock to which it is attached.

Treatment   Torn muscles heal well when repaired surgically, provided any dead tissue is removed and infection controlled.

Tendons heal slowly as they have a very poor blood supply and the repair can easily break down after the ends have been sutured together. It is necessary therefore for the dog to be completely rested after surgery and if a large tendon such as the Achilles tendon is involved, the leg is usually supported in a cast. Tendon repair is normally achieved using stainless steel, nylon, or more recently developed slowly dissolving sutures.

Infections

Muscle infection usually arises from a penetrating wound, such as a dog bite or stick injury. The muscle becomes hot and painful and if the infection is severe, the dog may be depressed and off his food. An abscess may form and discharge pus through the skin at the site of the original injury.

Treatment   The wound should be bathed with sterile saline and antibiotics may be prescribed by the vet. In severe cases, it may be necessary to remove any diseased tissue surgically and to insert a drainage tube to effect mechanical drainage of pus from the wound.

Myositis of the Jaw Muscles

The cause of this acute, painful inflammation of the jaw muscles is not known. The muscles become swollen and the dog will be reluctant to open his mouth.

Treatment   Pain-killing and/or anti-inflammatory drugs usually help but, if the condition is severe, some of the muscle fibres will be replaced by scar tissue and the muscles appear wasted. Contraction of this scar tissue makes it difficult for the dog to open his mouth. Once scar tissue has formed, treatment is unsuccessful so affected dogs should be encouraged to chew on bones during the early stages of the disease in order to discourage this scar tissue formation.

Atrophy

Atrophy means wasting and muscles waste if they are not used or if the nerve supply is damaged. A dog with a long-standing, severe lameness loses muscle bulk on the affected limb but this loss is reversible if the muscles start to function normally again. Physiotherapy helps to prevent atrophy by encouraging movement of the muscles.

However, if the muscle wastage is due to permanent damage to the nerve supply to that muscle, it is not reversible. The muscle wastes slowly over many weeks and then starts to contract, resulting in fixation of the limb. Muscle wastage and loss of limb function, in our experience, occurs most commonly following a road traffic accident in which a blow to the shoulder damages the radial nerve. The resulting radial paralysis causes a total dysfunction of the affected leg which, because it is paralysed, is merely dragged along by the dog. If the blow is not severe, the use returns to the leg over a period of days or weeks but, if the damage to the nerve was total, the paralysis is permanent and the leg will contract and stiffen. Surgical amputation is usually necessary in such cases and the patient adapts extremely well. The abnormal contracted limb is a hindrance to the dog and his mobility is considerably increased once it has been removed.

13 The Nervous System

The nervous system is the most complicated system in the body and the one that is the most difficult to understand. Its function is to regulate all the other body systems and to receive information about the outside world which it relays to the brain. The brain then analyses this information and decides if any action needs to be taken. Messages are then relayed back along nerves to organs that will carry out that action or function.

NORMAL STRUCTURE AND FUNCTION

The nervous system can be conveniently divided into two parts.

The central nervous system (CNS)   This system consists of the brain lying in the skull and the spinal cord which runs from the brain through the spinal canal within the backbone or vertebral column.

The peripheral nervous system (PNS)
This system comprises the nerves which connect the CNS to all the organs of the body, such as the skin, heart and muscles.

The Brain

The major parts of the brain are the cerebrum, cerebellum and brainstem. The cerebrum controls conscious thought and actions, the cerebellum is responsible for the coordination of these actions, and the brainstem controls the vital functions of the body such as heartbeat and respiration. All these structures are hollow and filled with a circulating fluid, the cerebrospinal fluid (CSF), which supplies the brain with additional nutrients.

The Nerve Cell

The basic units of the nervous system are the millions of tiny nerve cells, called neurones. Each neurone consists of a cell body from

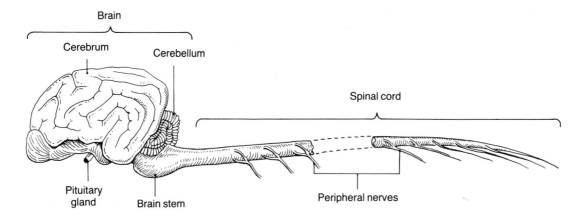

Fig 34 Central Nervous System

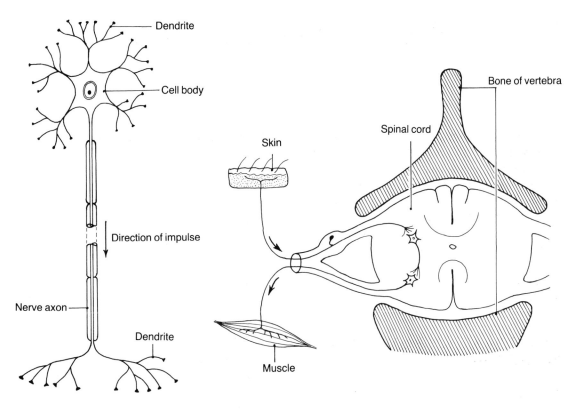

Fig 35 A typical nerve cell (neurone), greatly magnified

which arises a long process called an axon. Both ends of the nerve cell divide into very fine processes called dendrites. These dendrites make contact with dendrites from other nerve cells and the area of contact is called a synapse. When a nerve cell 'fires', an electrical impulse passes down the axon and when it reaches the synapse at the end, a chemical is released which passes across the synapse and activates the next nerve cell. Nerve tissue is very soft and any pressure on a nerve axon will reduce the ability of that nerve to transmit an impulse. Complete compression of the axon will render that nerve functionless (paralysed).

Types of Nerve

There are two main types of nerve in the nervous system – sensory nerves and motor nerves. Sensory nerves pass messages *to* the brain *from* sensory organs, such as the eye or skin, whereas motor nerves pass messages *from* the brain *to* the receiving organs, such as the muscles. In the central nervous system, the motor and sensory nerves follow different pathways but within the peripheral nerves they run side by side.

Reflexes

A nerve reflex is an automatic response to a certain stimulus which enables the CNS to carry out many functions without conscious thought. Much clinical information about the proper functioning of the nervous system can be gained from the study of these reflexes. A reflex simply consists of a sensory nerve which arises from a sensor in, for instance, the skin or tendon and ends in a specific area of the CNS, such as the spinal cord. The reflex arc is completed when the message is relayed through a short connecting nerve to a motor nerve and then to a muscle. The knee jerk is an example of a simple reflex. When the muscle above the knee is slightly stretched by tapping the tendon below the knee, stretch sensors in the muscle fire and an impulse passes along a sensory nerve to the lower part of the spinal cord. The impulse, instead of passing to the brain, passes along a connecting nerve to the motor nerve which stimulates the muscle to contract so bringing the leg back to the original position. If this reflex fails, the vet knows there is damage to either the nerves of the hind leg or the lower part of the spinal cord. There are reflexes in almost every part of the nervous system.

Some small nerves, called the autonomic nerves, supply the internal organs of the body. They control such organs as the eye, the heart and digestive system which are not under the conscious control of the brain.

DISEASES OF THE BRAIN

Bacterial Infection

Bacterial infections of the brain are rare in the dog. They cause meningitis, which is an inflammation of the covering membranes, the meninges. Bacteria enter the brain through penetrating wounds of the skull, ear infections or via the blood from other areas of infection in the body.

An affected dog is lethargic, off his food and has a raised temperature. He is reluctant to move, seeks dark areas and may show stiffness of the neck.

Diagnosis This can be difficult and may require laboratory testing of blood and cerebrospinal fluid.

Treatment Specific antibiotics are used in high doses but the prognosis is poor.

Tetanus

Dirty wounds may become infected with the tetanus bacteria, *Clostridium tetani*, which multiply and produce toxins in the wound. These toxins travel along the nerves from the wound to the CNS where they stimulate the motor nerves, so causing spasm of the muscles. Dogs are normally very resistant to tetanus and, in most cases, may show simply a stiffness of the tail and a 'tightness' of the facial muscles. The full disease syndrome with severe muscular spasms, lockjaw and death is rarely seen in dogs.

Diagnosis This is normally based on the clinical signs.

Treatment Patients must be kept quiet and treated with tetanus antitoxin, antibiotics and sedative drugs. This disease is so uncommon in dogs, unlike in man or horses, that it is not necessary to vaccinate them against it.

Viral Infections

Viruses can attack and destroy brain cells, causing encephalitis. The two most important diseases involving viruses which cause encephalitis are canine distemper and rabies discussed in greater detail in Chapter 5 (*see* pages 61 and 70). Symptoms of viral encephalitis vary greatly from paralysis to fits, depending on which brain cells are affected.

Diagnosis This is based on the clinical signs, but laboratory testing may be necessary.

Treatment There is no specific treatment available for viral encephalitis, but supportive therapy such as antibiotics to prevent secondary infection and sedatives to reduce convulsions, may be necessary. The patient should be kept under quiet, calm conditions, preferably in a darkened room.

Trauma (Damage)

The dog's brain is very well protected from damage by the thick skull and the fact that the brain is relatively small. However, damage to the brain can occur in two ways:

Localised trauma

A small part of the brain may be damaged by, for example, a small depressed fracture of the skull and the symptoms shown will depend on the part of the brain affected. For example, blindness may occur if the visual part of the brain is affected, or the dog may be paralysed on one side if the motor cortex is damaged.

Generalised trauma

As brain tissue is very soft and encased in a rigid box, the skull, any damage resulting in swelling of the brain (oedema) and haemorrhage will apply pressure to the soft brain tissue. Severe bruising or oedema of the brain will result in loss of consciousness. However, less severe damage will produce a dull, weak dog who will have difficulty in moving and lose interest in food and water. His pupils may be widely dilated and seizures or fits may develop. This swelling of the brain can cause concussion.

Diagnosis A diagnosis may be made from the clinical signs and a history of trauma or evidence of a fractured skull, although radiography may be required.

Treatment This must be instigated immediately to prevent permanent damage. Drugs are used to reduce the oedema and the dog must be kept quiet. Sedatives may be given to prevent seizures or struggling. Depressed fractures require surgical repair. Recovery from brain damage can take a long time and it may be impossible for the vet to predict how long or how complete the recovery will be after his initial examination. As shock is invariably involved, treatment for this is given as outlined in Chapter 18 (see page 216).

Hydrocephalus

Hydrocephalus is a condition caused by an increase in CSF pressure within the chambers of the brain and leads to pressure damage to the brain cells. Most cases are congenital but some are caused by disease processes such as tumours, which obstruct the flow of CSF. The increase in pressure can be so severe that only a narrow rim of normal brain tissue remains.

Clinical signs include dullness, weakness and fits.

Diagnosis This is based on the clinical signs, the dome-shape appearance of the head and can be confirmed by measuring the CSF pressure on needle puncture of the spinal canal.

Treatment There is no satisfactory treatment but some puppies with mild hydrocephalus will adapt and lead a fairly normal life.

Vestibular Syndrome

This is a fairly common condition of the older dog in which the area of the brain which controls balance is affected on one side. The onset is sudden. Symptoms include a head tilt to the affected side, the dog may fall or circle to that side and there is a flicking movement of the eyes, called

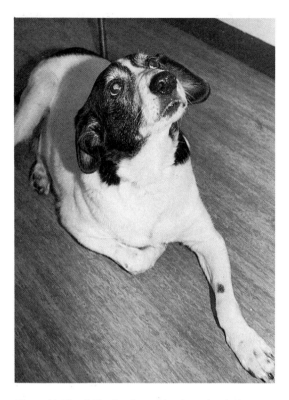

Dog with Vestibular Syndrome showing a head tilt to the right.

nystagmus. There may also be vomiting in the initial stages of the disease. The severity of the condition varies, some dogs being unable to stand while others are hardly affected. Many dogs will recover slowly in about five days but this condition will often recur and may be more severe the next time. Vestibular syndrome can be caused by cerebrovascular spasm (constriction of the blood vessel in the brain), a localised brain infection or disease of the inner ear. This syndrome is often referred to as a 'stroke' although it is not identical to the disease in man.

Poisons

Poisons which affect the CNS are not encountered frequently but the four most common are described below.

Lead Poisoning

This condition usually occurs in puppies as they are more likely to chew unusual objects. Common sources of lead are old paint, lead piping, old batteries and linoleum. Lead poisoning produces a whole range of clinical signs but initially those of a gastrointestinal upset, vomiting, diarrhoea and colic. Later CNS signs develop which may include fits, blindness, over-excitement and behavioural changes.

Lead poisoning is diagnosed in the laboratory by raised blood lead levels.

Treatment The lead can be removed from the body by injecting a drug, sodium calcium edetate, which combines with the lead, enabling it to be excreted through the kidneys.

Slug bait Poisoning (Metaldehyde)

If a dog eats enough slug bait to cause CNS disturbances, he will initially appear drunk but sometimes, this incoordination progresses and leads to the inability to stand and a loss of consciousness. Convulsions occur in extreme cases.

Treatment There is no specific antidote but if the dog has recently swallowed the metaldehyde, he can be given an emetic to make him vomit and empty the stomach. If severe neurological signs develop, the dog will require intravenous sedatives and fluid therapy. In the experience of the authors, most dogs will not normally eat enough metaldehyde to cause death. Nevertheless, slug bait poisoning is considered to be a veterinary emergency.

Strychnine Poisoning

This is now very rare as strychnine is virtually unobtainable. However, it causes complete paralysis with spasms which increase when the dog is subjected to noise. There is no antidote and the dog must be kept quiet and sedated to prevent spasms. Death nearly always ensues.

Alphachloralose (Pigeon and Mouse Poison)

This poison acts by reducing the body temperature and can cause profound depression. Sometimes, however, it causes excitation with fits.

Treatment   There is no specific antidote, but the vast majority of dogs recover, provided attention is paid to keeping them very warm.

Inherited Disease

There are many inherited diseases which cause a whole range of neurological symptoms including blindness, incoordination, tremors, weakness and poor growth. The symptoms occur in puppies aged between about four weeks and one year and therefore are discussed in Chapter 4, The Growing Dog (*see* page 53).

Convulsions, Seizures or Fits

A seizure occurs when some brain cells, which are functioning abnormally, fire spontaneously and this activity quickly spreads through the surrounding brain. A seizure which is localised to one part of the brain is called a petit mal seizure; if it affects the whole brain, it is called a grand mal seizure.

Petit mal seizures can produce a whole range of signs. Sometimes, the dog may just stand still and shake for a very short period, one leg may twitch, his personality may change, or he may just bark uncontrollably for a while. Imaginary fly-catching in Cavalier King Charles Spaniels is thought to be a petit mal seizure.

A grand mal seizure usually occurs when the animal is at rest. The dog falls onto his side, his legs become rigid and move with paddling movements, his eyes are open and staring and his lips are drawn back. Usually he makes a chewing action with his jaws and salivates excessively. He may also defaecate and urinate. Most fits last for no more than two to five minutes. When the fit subsides, the dog will be unsteady and confused but within half an hour he will usually be back to normal. Occasionally a fit will become continuous, a condition known as status epilepticus.

Action   During a fit the owner must reduce any unnecessary extraneous noise such as the radio or television, reduce the light in the room and prevent the dog from damaging himself. If he has fallen into an awkward position, it may be necessary to move him to an open space during a fit and this is most effectively carried out by dragging him gently by his hind legs. Do not attempt to pull the tongue out or to sit the dog up.

There are several causes of fits, listed below.

Primary Epilepsy

Primary epilepsy has no known cause but it does occur more frequently in certain breeds, especially the German Shepherd Dog and the Golden Retriever. The first fit usually occurs when the dog is one to two years old. The fits increase in frequency until in some cases they can occur several times a week.

The diagnosis of primary epilepsy is based on the type of fit, the age and breed of dog and the elimination of other possible causes.

Infections

Any infection which damages the brain cells can cause convulsions. In the dog, one of the most common is canine distemper where the fits may develop months or even years after the initial infection. Once fits have started there is usually no cure.

Trauma

Trauma may cause convulsions by damaging brain cells. Diagnosis is based on the history of trauma to the head or spine and the elimination of other diseases.

Tumours

Small tumours will sometimes produce convulsions but, in most cases, as the tumour grows, other neurological signs will develop as well.

Metabolic disease

Diseases of other organs may alter the blood levels of substances which will affect the brain. Certain liver and kidney diseases, for instance, can increase the level of toxic substances in the blood. Disease of the pancreas can reduce blood sugar and severe respiratory disease can produce a very low blood oxygen level. Low blood calcium can result from diseases of the parathyroid glands, or occur during milk fever. These various causes of seizures are diagnosed by laboratory testing of blood samples and, in most cases, if the underlying disease can be treated successfully, the fits will cease.

Treatment   There are many anti-epileptic drugs available but treatment with them is not straightforward as the effectiveness of different drugs and dosages can vary greatly from dog to dog. Sometimes, anti-convulsant drugs will be used in combination, but the general aim of treatment is to prevent a fit without sedating the dog. Once treatment has started, it must not be stopped without advice from your vet or a fit may be precipitated.

DISEASES OF THE SPINAL CORD

Diseases of the spinal cord nearly always start as a weakness and incoordination of the limbs, especially the hind legs. If the damage is in the neck then usually, but not always, all four legs are affected. If the damage occurs between front and rear legs then only the rear legs and tail are affected.

Inherited Diseases

The Wobbler Syndrome

This disease is caused by a deformity of the bones in the neck (the cervical vertebrae) and is mostly seen in the Dobermann, Setters and Great Dane. The age of onset varies between six months and eight years although it peaks at around two years. The deformity of the vertebrae results in narrowing of the spinal canal with resultant pressure on the spinal cord. Although the lesion is in the neck, the longer nerves are at most risk and so symptoms are first seen in the hind legs. Incoordination and weakness slowly progress until the dog has difficulty getting up and has a 'wobbly' hind leg gait.

Treatment   This is diagnosed by the presence of the deformed vertebrae on a neck X-ray. Some dogs will improve with rest and anti-inflammatory treatment, but most will require disc fenestration (an operation to remove the contents of an intervertebral disc) or an operation to fuse the affected vertebrae in the correct position. This fusion is normally carried out using bone screws, and prevents movement of the deformed bones and the resulting pressure on the spinal cord.

Hemivertebrae

This is a rare condition of the brachycephalic (short-nosed) breeds, especially those with screw tails – the Bulldog and the Boston Terrier. The individual vertebrae are deformed and by causing narrowing of the spinal canal, they apply pressure to the spinal cord. The symptoms of weakness and incoordination develop at about three months of age and are often progressive. Diagnosis is by an X-ray of the spine. There is no treatment for this condition.

Atlanto-Axial Dislocation

In this condition, seen in the young of toy breeds especially Yorkies, there is a deformity between the first and second cervical vertebrae in the neck, which results in intermittent pressure on the spinal cord. The symptoms include neck pain, sudden collapse and sometimes weakness and incoordination of the hind legs.

The deformity can be seen on an X-ray of the neck vertebrae.

Treatment   There is no effective medical treatment but surgical fusion of the two vertebrae in the correct position, using bone screws, can alleviate the symptoms.

Chronic Degenerative Radiculomyelopathy (CDRM)

This is a fairly common syndrome in some large breeds of dog, especially the German Shepherd Dog. Usually dogs are over six years of age when they begin to show symptoms and both sexes can be affected.

The cause of CDRM is not known but some nerve tracts and nerve roots in the spinal cord begin to degenerate and their ability to conduct nerve impulses is impaired. It is always progressive but usually slow in onset and the first sign may just be a slight weakness of the hind legs. This slowly progresses to ataxia, or swaying of the hind legs, with a peculiar high-stepping walk, then crossing of the hind legs and dragging of the hind feet with wearing down of the nails as the paralysis progresses. At no stage is there any pain.

Your veterinary surgeon will diagnose the condition based on the breed, the clinical symptoms and, possibly, the absence of other diseases on X-ray.

Treatment   There is no effective treatment although anabolic or cortico-steroids occasionally seem to slow down the progress of the disease.

Eventually, the patient loses the use of the hind legs completely and, at this stage or just before, euthanasia is usually recommended on humane grounds.

Trauma

The spinal cord is well protected in the spinal canal by the surrounding vertebrae and so damage to it is uncommon. Most spinal cord injuries are caused by road accidents but occasionally a severe back sprain will lead to damage. There are two different forms of trauma to the cord which cannot always be easily differentiated on initial examination:

Complete Rupture of the Spinal Cord

The spinal cord can be completely severed so that there can be no nerve transmission across the break. The limbs behind the lesion will be completely paralysed and there can be no recovery. This type of injury caused by a broken spine is nearly always the result of a road traffic accident. Usually the break occurs in the mid-spine between the fore and hind legs. The dog will be in a lot of pain and unable to move the affected legs.

Treatment   A pain-killer, sedative or

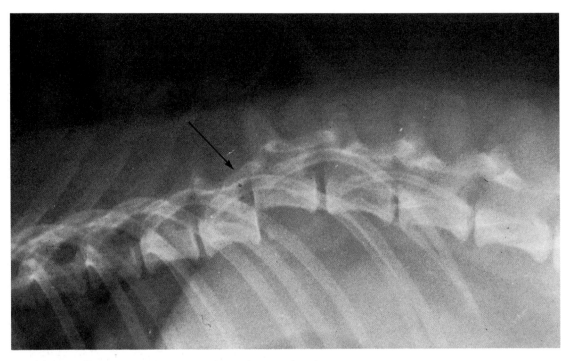

An X-ray of a fractured spine with complete rupture of the spinal cord.

anaesthetic is administered to allow a full examination and the fractured spine can be seen on X-ray. As the pain is so severe, and as there is no chance of recovery, it is advisable to euthanase the dog immediately to prevent further suffering.

Bruising of the Spine

The spinal cord has a large blood supply and, in less severe accidents, the spine may remain intact but its blood vessels may be ruptured. As the cord is enclosed in a bony tube, any haemorrhage will fill the space and exert pressure on the nerves. The clinical signs depend on the degree of haemorrhage and the site of the injury and they range from weakness to total paralysis. There is usually far less pain than in a case of spinal fracture. An X-ray of the spinal cord will differentiate between a broken back and spinal bruising although contrast radiography may be needed to locate the haemorrhage.

Treatment Surgery to remove the blood clot is rarely attempted but drugs are administered to reduce this pressure on the nerves. The dog must be kept quiet to prevent further damage and it may be necessary to catheterise and empty the bladder which may also be paralysed.

The outcome of treatment of these injuries is very difficult to predict but, in general, the more severe the clinical signs, the less favourable the outcome.

Prolapsed Intervertebral Disc

This is a common condition of the small breeds, especially the Dachshund with his long back. Each intervertebral disc forms a cushion between two vertebrae and consists of a soft jelly-like centre, enclosed by a fibrous band. Unfortunately, this fibrous band is thinnest just below the spinal cord so when a disc ruptures, the jelly-like centre is squeezed upwards against the spinal cord and nerves, applying pressure and causing

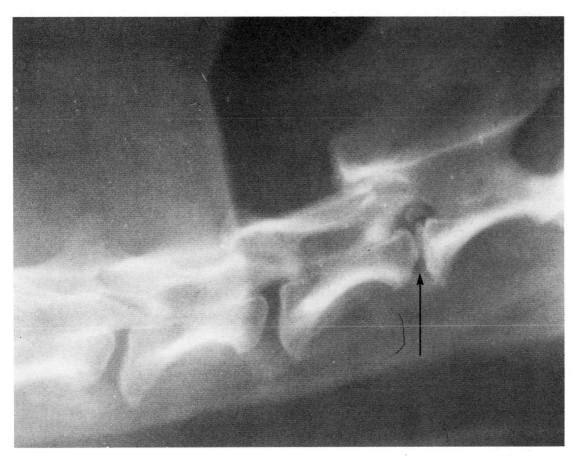

A prolapsed calcified intervertebral disc in the neck.

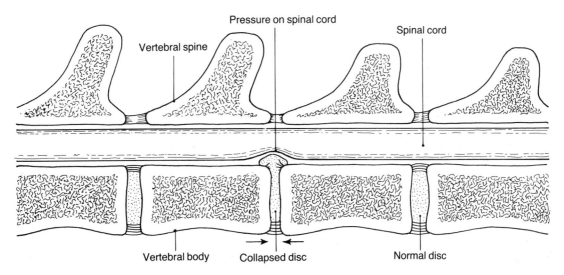

Fig 36 Section of the spinal cord showing a collapsed disc

inflammation. The two most common loc-ations for disc disease are in the neck (cervical) and in the midback (thoraco-lumbar), where the thoracic vertebrae meet the lumbar vertebrae. Disc disease is usually seen in the middle-aged dog due to the disc finally rupturing after much wear and tear.

Collapse of the cervical disc tends to produce pain symptoms rather than signs of nerve damage. The dog holds his neck very stiffly, is reluctant to eat or move and will howl if the neck is manipulated. Very often, the slightest movement will cause the dog to cry out. Only in severe cases will typical signs of nerve damage also be present.

Damage to the thoraco-lumbar discs produces a greater variety of symptoms. Mild damage to the disc produces back pain with no nerve dysfunction and, therefore, no lameness. The dog is quiet and may have a hunched back. He is reluctant to climb steps or jump, is often off his food and cries when picked up. As the disc collapses more into the spinal canal, the increased pressure will start to affect nerve function. Clinical signs vary from a slight incoordination to complete hind leg paralysis, with loss of bladder and bowel function.

Diagnosis The clinical signs coupled with pain on examination of the spine can be diagnostic. An X-ray will confirm this, as most collapsed discs will show as a narrowed space between the vertebrae. However, in some cases, pressure on the spinal cord can only be demonstrated by contrast myelo-graphy (the introduction of a radio-opaque dye into the spinal canal).

Treatment The vast majority of cases of prolapsed discs will respond to medical treatment which is aimed at reducing the inflammation and swelling around the disc. The dog must be confined in a small space and in cases where this function is lost, the bladder must be emptied. Some dogs, especially those with recurrent pain, will require spinal surgery to remove the affected disc, and where this is necessary, surgical treatment is normally carried out as soon as possible after the onset of signs.

Unfortunately, not all dogs with disc problems recover and some are left with completely paralysed hind legs. The owner of a permanently paralysed dog has the choice of euthanasia, or providing a 'wheelchair'. One manufacturer makes an orthopaedic wheeled support for the hind legs which enables the dog to move around freely. Not all dogs can adapt to this and the incontinence problem still remains. We have seen successes, though, especially where the patient is a young small active dog.

Tumours

Tumours of the spinal cord are rare. The symptoms seen are caused by pressure on the nerves producing incoordination and weak-ness in one or more legs, depending on the site of the tumour. Usually the tumour can be seen on an X-ray, with or without myelography. Unfortunately, there is no successful treatment for spinal tumours and euthanasia is normally the treatment chosen.

DISEASES OF THE PERIPHERAL NERVES

Damage to the peripheral nerves can cause loss of reflexes, paralysis of the affected limb or loss of feeling.

Trauma

Peripheral nerves are rarely damaged by trauma, which is surprising when one considers the frequency of bone fractures. The nerve most commonly affected is the radial nerve which supplies the front leg. This nerve can be damaged by a blow to the shoulder area and, when this occurs, the leg will hang loosely at the dog's side and will be unable to bear weight. The dog will drag the leg when he walks. There is no sensation in the leg and no pain. This injury is frequently mistaken by the owner for a broken leg.

Treatment There is no specific treatment for radial nerve paralysis but drugs which reduce inflammation may be helpful. Unfortunately it is not always possible to assess the degree of damage and only time will tell if nerve function will return. If the leg remains paralysed, there will be severe muscle wastage and contraction, with sores developing on those parts of the leg which drag on the ground. If the paralysis is permanent, the leg, in addition to being of no use to the dog, is often a hindrance so amputation is usually advised.

Horner's Syndrome

This is a condition of sudden onset which affects one eye causing a dilated pupil, a dropped upper lid and a protruding third eyelid. There is no apparent effect on eyesight. Horner's syndrome is caused when the nerve which supplies the eye and eyelids is damaged. Ear infections, tumours or trauma can damage this nerve as it leaves the spinal cord between the thoracic vertebrae in the chest and runs up the neck past the inner ear to the eye. In many cases, the cause remains a mystery.

Treatment Many cases recover spontaneously although some persist. Anti-inflammatory treatment may help.

Facial Paralysis

This is a rare condition which affects the nerve supplying the facial muscles (the muscles which move the lips, nose and eyelids). The paralysis is usually on one side and signs include drooping of the lips and eyelids, and a deviation of the nose to the unaffected side. There is often no obvious cause but a blow to the nerve as it crosses the side of the face is often postulated.

Treatment Anti-inflammatory drugs may help but facial paralysis is often permanent.

Myasthenia Gravis

This is a rare condition which affects the motor nerves where they supply the muscles. An affected dog has a very low exercise tolerance and after a short period of exercise, he collapses. After a little rest he continues his exercise only to collapse again.

Diagnosis and treatment The disease is diagnosed by giving a trial injection of a drug which aids transmission between nerve and muscle and thus increases the length of time the dog can be exercised if he suffers from myasthenia gravis. If this test proves positive, myasthenia gravis is treated with a similar drug in tablet form.

Botulism

Toxins are released from *Clostridium botulinum* bacteria in rotting carcasses, especially those of waterbirds, and dogs become affected by botulism by eating this rotten meat. It can also occur as a contaminant in damaged cans of meat or fish. An affected dog becomes completely paralysed and unable to move.

Treatment There is no specific treatment, but patients are fed by intravenous fluid therapy until recovery occurs. If enough toxins are ingested to affect the nerves supplying the respiratory muscles, the dog may die from respiratory failure.

14 The Urinary System

The urinary system comprises two kidneys and ureters and a single bladder and urethra. Its function is to maintain the correct composition of body fluids and to control the excretion of waste products from the body. These are formed mainly from the breakdown of food, especially excess protein, but also from the natural breakdown of body tissues such as muscle.

NORMAL STRUCTURE AND FUNCTION

The kidneys are situated in the upper part of the abdomen, on either side, and they lie below the back muscles. The right kidney lies slightly in front of the left and both can normally be palpated by the vet in a thin dog. Each kidney is composed of numerous

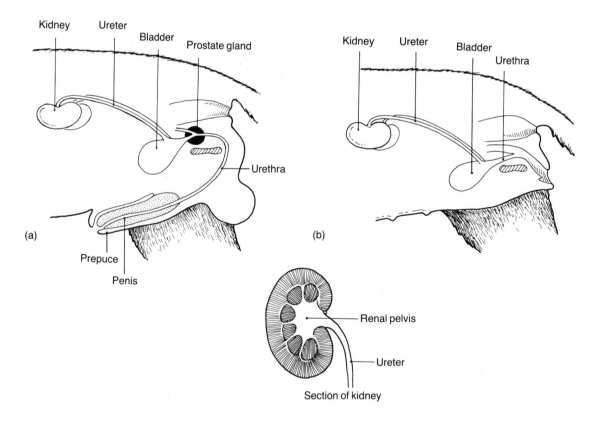

Fig 37 (a) Urinary system of the male dog
(b) Urinary system of the bitch

little tubes, called nephrons. The nephrons first filter the blood and then, as the resulting fluid passes along the tube, they concentrate it to produce urine. This process of filtration is regulated by the release of hormones from the brain and requires a large blood supply. Urine consists of waste nitrogenous products, mainly urea and other waste substances, excess body water and minerals. The kidney also produces hormones itself which affect blood pressure and red blood cell production. The urine collects in a part of the kidney called the renal pelvis and then leaves each kidney through a very fine tube, the ureter. The two ureters run through the abdomen and enter the neck of the bladder.

The bladder is an expandable, muscular sac lying on the floor of the abdomen, just in front of the pelvis. Urine is expelled into the urethra by contraction of the bladder and abdominal muscles. The small nerves which control bladder function arise from the spinal cord, at the level of the pelvis and run through the pelvic canal to the bladder wall. These nerves are easily damaged by injury to this area.

The urethra is a narrow, muscular tube through which urine is expelled from the bladder. In the bitch, the urethra is short and runs through the pelvis under the rectum to enter the vulva behind the vagina. However, in the male dog the urethra is much longer. It runs backwards through the pelvis but then passes forwards above the scrotum and into the penis. Within the penis lies a small bone, the os penis, which has a groove in which the urethra passes to the tip of the penis.

Correct functioning of the urinary system is necessary for the maintenance of life and, therefore, any disease affecting this system is potentially life threatening. Human medicine has made great advances in the treatment of kidney disease in recent years, with the development of artificial kidneys and kidney transplants. Unfortunately, in general practice, veterinary medicine does not yet aspire to these advanced treatments. The techniques are available but the inconveniences to the dog and the costs mean that advances are slow.

DISEASES PRODUCING AN INCREASED THIRST

Acute Kidney Failure (Acute Nephritis)

Acute kidney failure is an inflammation of the kidney leading to failure of urine production and, if severe, will rapidly produce a sick dog. The important clinical signs are lethargy, loss of appetite, abdominal pain and vomiting. In the early stages of acute nephritis, little urine is produced because swelling of the nephrons blocks the filtration process. However, as damage to the nephrons continues, large quantities of dilute urine are produced. Therefore, during the first few days of acute kidney failure there is little change in water intake but the thirst increases when the damage to the nephrons has been established.

Causes of acute kidney failure include:

Infection

The most important infectious agent producing acute nephritis is a bacterium called *Leptospira canicola* (see Chapter 5); infected dog urine is the main source. This disease is prevented by routine vaccination and so is not often seen. Apart from the clinical signs already mentioned, the dog will have a temperature of 40–41°C (104–106°F), and will usually be unvaccinated or will be overdue a booster vaccination.

Diagnosis This is usually made on clinical signs but blood tests can help. The organism can also be isolated from the urine in the laboratory.

175

Treatment Leptospirosis responds to treatment with antibiotics and, if the disease is treated in the early stages, there will often be a complete recovery with little residual damage to the kidneys. However, a prolonged infection will produce severe kidney scarring and lead to chronic kidney failure, called chronic interstitial nephritis. A light diet of high quality protein or reduced protein should be fed. Ideal prescription diets are available from your vet.

Failure of Urine Flow

Acute kidney failure will develop if there is a complete blockage of urine flow, which results in back pressure on the nephrons. The two most common causes are blockage of the urinary tract with a calculus or stone, and paralysis of the bladder following loss of nerve function. This nerve paralysis can occur following a prolapsed intervertebral disc or a fractured pelvis or spine.

Shock

Shock will lead to acute kidney failure because the blood pressure falls to such a low level that the filtration process in the nephrons ceases. The main causes of shock are severe accidents, especially road accidents, profuse haemorrhage and fluid-losing diseases such as parvovirus. Occasionally, blood pressure will fall during a major operation thus affecting the kidney and so slowing post-operative recovery. Kidney failure may only become apparent several days after the initial injury. To avoid acute kidney failure, shock is treated as soon as possible by restoring blood pressure with intravenous fluid therapy and using appropriate intravenous drugs.

Toxins and Poisons

Many poisons such as paraquat (weed killer) and antifreeze can rapidly damage the kidney to produce the typical signs of acute kidney failure. As most of these poisons have no specific antidote, treatment is directed at flushing out the poison by intravenous fluid therapy and supporting kidney function with drugs and special low protein diets.

Toxins released from bacteria which cause severe infections such as large abscesses, gastroenteritis and uterine infections can cause acute kidney failure. In such cases, it is important to treat the underlying disease. For example, an abscess must be drained or a very toxic uterus removed surgically. In most cases, kidney function will return to normal once the toxic cause is eliminated.

Chronic Kidney Failure

This is a common condition of old dogs but it is also seen occasionally in younger animals. Chronic kidney failure occurs when persistent damage to the kidney reduces the number of functional nephrons to a level at which the kidney cannot perform its proper function. This allows toxic substances, such as urea, to accumulate in the circulation. When urea is present in significant quantities in the blood the animal is said to be uraemic. In the old dog, chronic kidney failure results from repeated kidney infections. In the young dog, the cause is usually a congenital abnormality of the kidney.

The first signs of chronic renal failure are an increased frequency and volume of urination with a concurrent increase in thirst and a gradual weight loss. As the disease progresses and the blood urea rises, the dog becomes lethargic and his appetite starts to fail. The owner may notice an unpleasant mouth odour due to uraemia and associated gum and mouth ulcers. In some cases, the patient's bones may become very soft, due to the excessive loss of minerals. The dog will become anaemic which adds to his lethargy. In the final stages of the disease there is a complete loss of appetite, persistent vomiting, and extreme weakness, followed by convulsions, coma and death.

Diagnosis A diagnosis of chronic renal failure is confirmed by testing urine for protein loss and specific gravity, and blood for blood urea levels.

Treatment The prognosis is poor as chronic renal failure is irreversible and treatment is aimed at maximising the function of any remaining kidney tissue. Water must be available at all times and, where a patient is dehydrated, it may be necessary to replace fluid by intravenous therapy. Rest is important, stress should be avoided and special diets rich in energy and low in protein must be fed. Ideal canned or dry prescription diets are available from your vet. Anabolic steroids may be prescribed to help prevent weight loss.

In a normal dog, as in a human, one kidney can be removed safely without threatening life. In fact, a dog can live normally even if his total kidney tissue is reduced by some seventy-five per cent of its normal amount. Therefore, in chronic kidney failure, there may be sufficient kidney function to maintain a relatively fit animal. However, if this residual kidney tissue is suddenly stressed by, for example, a road accident or superimposed infection, kidney function may completely fail. The result is a very ill dog, showing all the typical signs of acute kidney failure including lethargy, a poor appetite and vomiting. Treatment of such a patient is often unsuccessful because the kidney reserves have already been destroyed. The dog will require intensive treatment from the vet, including intravenous fluid therapy and hospitalisation but despite all this, he is unlikely to recover.

Tumours

Tumours of the kidneys are rare and if both are affected, kidney failure will result. The most common tumour to develop in both kidneys is a lymphosarcoma and the disease pattern will be similar to that of chronic renal failure. There is no treatment.

If a single kidney is affected by a tumour, the signs will be those of abdominal enlargement and discomfort. Diagnosis is by palpation and radiography, and the tumour and affected kidney can be removed surgically in an operation called a nephrectomy. If the tumour is not malignant, the dog should recover well and function normally on his remaining kidney.

Diabetes Insipidus

Diabetes insipidus is an uncommon condition in which there is failure of the pituitary gland in the brain to produce a hormone which controls the kidney's ability to concentrate urine. Without this hormone, the kidney produces vast quantities of dilute urine and so the dog drinks more (up to five litres a day) to replenish fluid loss.

Diagnosis This is based on clinical symptoms, and by testing the specific gravity of urine and the ability of the dog to concentrate it.

Treatment The use of certain drugs will sometimes control the excess thirst and urination.

DISEASES PRODUCING BLOOD IN THE URINE

Pyelonephritis

Pyelonephritis is a disease characterised by an accumulation of pus within the kidney. The infection usually reaches the renal pelvis by ascending the ureter from the bladder. The symptoms, similar to those of acute nephritis, are a raised temperature, poor appetite, abdominal pain and vomiting. Blood and pus may also be seen in the urine.

Diagnosis This is based on the symptoms and confirmed by laboratory testing of blood and urine.

Treatment A prolonged course of the appropriate antibiotic is needed to treat this condition but the kidneys may be permanently damaged and chronic renal failure is a possible sequel. Attention to diet is important to avoid stressing the kidneys and a light diet, or prescription diet from your vet, should be fed. The dog should be encouraged to drink as much water as possible to flush the infection through.

Cystitis

Cystitis is the name given to inflammation of the bladder and is usually caused by an ascending infection from the urethra. It is seen more frequently in the bitch because the infection has easy access through the shorter urethra. The clinical signs include increased frequency of urination, straining and a bloody urine. In all other respects the dog usually appears healthy.

Diagnosis A diagnosis can often be made on clinical signs alone but urine tests are helpful when protein or blood can be detected. In addition, the causal bacteria can be identified and so the appropriate antibiotic can be prescribed.

Treatment Cystitis usually responds to a short course of antibiotics but it has a tendency to recur at frequent intervals in some dogs. These dogs may require repeated courses of antibiotics or constant treatment with urinary antiseptics or acidifiers to

prevent bacterial growth in the bladder. A low-grade chronic infection may result in a thick-walled bladder which requires long-term antibiotic treatment. However, some of these cases do not respond satisfactorily.

Bladder and Urethral Stones

Calculi or bladder stones are fairly common in both sexes in which they may present different clinical signs.

Bladder Stones

Calculi can irritate the bladder to produce cystitis and, in the bitch, this is usually the only clinical sign. The bitch will pass blood intermittently in the urine and there will be little or no response to antibiotic therapy. A male dog with large bladder stones may show very similar symptoms.

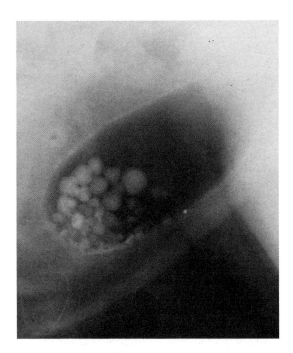

A urinary bladder, inflated with air, to show the presence of bladder stones or calculi.

Diagnosis Bladder stones can sometimes be detected when the vet palpates the dog's abdomen. They can be confirmed by X-raying the bladder, after gently filling it with air first which makes the stones easier to see.

Treatment There are several types of calculi. Depending on their chemical composition, some can be slowly dissolved by feeding the dog on a special diet, while others must be removed surgically. In some affected dogs there is a tendency for stones to recur but this can be prevented by the long-term use of prescription diets.

Urethral Stones

In the male dog, the most common initial sign is obstruction to urine flow, causing the dog to cock his leg and strain frequently and ineffectively. This is due to small calculi passing into the urethra and becoming lodged at the base of the bone in the penis where they cause obstruction. This leads to retention of urine and acute kidney failure ensues. Urethral obstruction is invariably seen in the male because of the much longer narrower urethra and the penile bone which prevents the urethra expanding to allow passage of the stone.

The initial clinical signs are those of acute abdominal discomfort with severe straining. A few drops of blood-tinged urine may be passed. If left untreated, the signs change to those of acute kidney failure – depression, inappetence and vomiting.

Treatment Urethral obstruction is an emergency situation and the dog should be taken to the vet for surgical removal of the offending stone without delay. Once the obstructing stone has been removed, the bladder can be examined for further calculi. If present, a cystotomy operation to remove them may be necessary.

Urethritis

Urethritis, or inflammation of the urethra, is usually caused by an ascending infection from the penis or vulva. It is often associated with cystitis and causes the same symptoms, although in the male, haemorrhage can be quite severe.

Treatment Urethritis is treated with antibiotics, the choice of which may depend on the result of the sensitivity testing of urine.

Tumours

Tumours of the bladder are uncommon, but when one occurs, the symptoms can appear in one of two ways. As in cystitis, there may be frequent straining and bloody urine due to the tumour eroding the inner lining of the bladder. The tumour may, on the other hand, damage the bladder wall rendering it

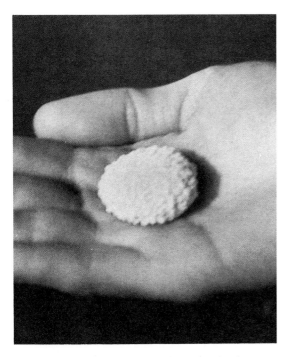

A bladder stone showing the irregular surface which can damage the bladder.

unable to contract normally. This will produce incontinence. Large tumours can often be felt by your vet through the abdominal wall or their presence can be detected on an X-ray.

Treatment Some bladder tumours can be treated with medical therapy or by surgical removal but most tumours in this area are not amenable to treatment.

DISEASES PRODUCING INCONTINENCE

Incontinence is the unconscious and uncontrolled leakage of urine from the urethra. It usually manifests as small puddles of urine whenever the dog lies down for any length of time. In some cases the leakage is continuous and obvious even when the dog walks. The hind legs become urine-stained. An offensive smell develops which is caused by the urine-soaked hair and infection of the urine-scalded skin.
    Causes of incontinence include:

Ectopic Ureters

An ectopic or misplaced ureter is a rare congenital condition of mainly female puppies who are born with usually one, but sometimes both, ureters entering the vagina instead of the bladder. As the bladder is bypassed, urine cannot be stored and so it constantly dribbles from the vulva. The problem usually becomes apparent once the puppy has left the nest and begins to move around the house.

Treatment Medical treatment is not effective and to cure the problem, the malpositioned ureter must be transplanted so that it enters the bladder instead of the vagina.

Hormonal Causes

Hormonal incontinence is an occasional problem of the larger spayed bitch and it usually occurs late in life. In our experience, it does not seem to be related to the age of spaying and in only a very few cases does the incontinence occur shortly after spaying.

Treatment Most patients respond to a short course of replacement hormone therapy and, although in most cases one course is enough, some bitches will need repeated treatments.

Short Urethra

Some bitches have a shorter urethra than normal and when extra pressure is exerted, urine may be forced out. In this case, surgery to anchor the bladder further forward in the abdomen, away from the pelvis, is often successful.

Lack of Uterine Ligaments

In the giant breeds especially, incontinence can be due to the bladder moving further back into the pelvis as the uterine ligaments which hold it in place are removed during the spay operation. In this case, surgery is needed to reposition the bladder further forward in the abdomen.

Nerve Damage

Any damage to the nerve supply to the bladder will lead to failure of urination and urine will accumulate until the bladder is full. Thereafter, urine will leak out at a rate equal to that of urine production. This incontinence of the paralysed bladder is an important clinical sign because it will produce firstly retention cystitis and then acute renal failure, due to back pressure on the kidneys.

This condition, as already mentioned, is most likely to result from a severe disc lesion or a fractured spine or pelvis.

Treatment   The bladder must be emptied either by manual pressure or preferably by the insertion of a catheter through the urethra. Treatment must be continued until bladder function returns.

Old Age

Senile incontinence occasionally occurs in aged dogs for no apparent reason. It is thought to be due to a gradual weakening of the sphincter muscle in the neck of the bladder. There is no treatment.

15 The Reproductive System

THE MALE DOG – NORMAL STRUCTURE AND FUNCTION

The functions of the male reproductive system are the production of semen, its introduction into the bitch's vagina, and the production of male hormones. The system is composed of paired testicles, each of which has an epididymis and a tube, the vas deferens; a single prostate gland; a urethra, and a penis with its protective sheath, the prepuce.

The testicles are oval in shape and lie in a sac, the scrotum, to keep them slightly below normal body temperature. They produce sperm and testosterone, the male hormone. This hormone, which enters the bloodstream, helps to determine male characteristics and behaviour. In the foetus the testicles are situated just behind the kidneys but, as the young puppy develops, they gradually move through an opening in the groin, the inguinal ring, until at about seven to ten days after birth, they come to lie in the scrotum.

The sperm leave each testicle through the vas deferens and enter the epididymis where they are stored. From here, on ejaculation, they enter the urethra just beyond the neck of the bladder. From this point the urethra is shared with the urinary system.

The prostate is a small gland which

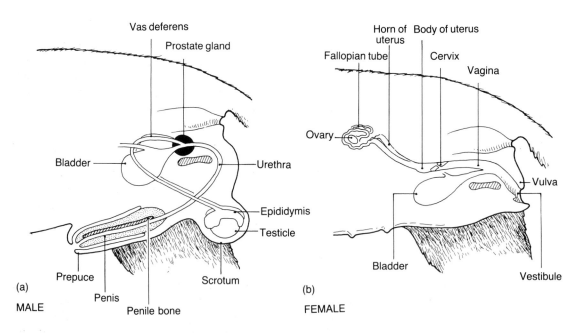

(a) MALE

(b) FEMALE

Fig 38 (a) Reproductive system of the male dog
(b) Reproductive system of the bitch

surrounds the urethra just behind the bladder in the pelvic canal. It produces a secretion which helps in the feeding and transport of the sperm.

The penis is enclosed in and protected by the prepuce and consists mostly of erectile tissue. At the base of the penis is a bulbous portion which swells during mating causing the male dog to become 'tied' with the bitch. In the penis of the dog is a bone, the os penis, through which the urethra runs.

DISEASES OF THE TESTICLES

Retained Testicle (Cryptorchidism)

Occasionally during development, one or both testicles may fail to descend into the scrotum and can be retained somewhere along their developmental path. However, as they can take a long time to descend, a definite diagnosis should be delayed until the dog is ten months old. The testicle is usually retained in one of two positions, either in the abdomen just inside the inguinal ring, or just outside the inguinal ring in the groin. In our experience, medical treatment to further the descent of these testicles into the scrotum is not successful. As the condition is considered to be hereditary, surgical correction is unethical. If carried out, it may lead to future generations of male dogs with the same condition. For the same reason, dogs which have one retained testicle should not be used for breeding.

Treatment Retained testicles are more susceptible to disease, especially cancerous change, and many vets will suggest surgical removal. The retained testicle, because it is at a higher temperature than normal, will not produce fertile sperm so a dog with both testicles retained is sterile.

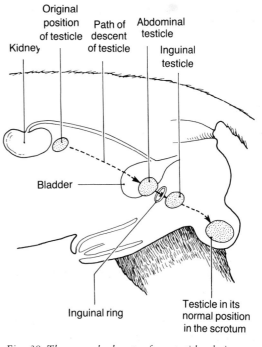

Fig 39 The normal descent of a testicle during development showing the main sites of retention

Orchitis

Orchitis or infection is very rare but when present, one or both testicles become very painful and swollen. An affected dog will usually have a raised temperature, refuse food and be reluctant to move.

Treatment Orchitis quickly responds to antibiotic therapy, but occasionally, an abscess may result which is much more resistant to treatment. In some cases, surgical removal of the affected testicle may be necessary.

Tumours

Tumours are fairly common but, fortunately, most are benign. They can become quite large and may interfere with walking. One type of testicular tumour, known as a Sertoli cell tumour, produces female hormones

183

which cause an affected dog to develop female characteristics. The teats and mammary glands enlarge and he becomes attractive to other male dogs. There may also be hair loss which begins symmetrically on each flank.

Treatment Once the tumourous testicle is removed, these changes invariably reverse, so surgery is the preferred treatment. It may be advisable to remove both testicles to eliminate the possibility of a recurrence.

Torsion

Very occasionally, especially where retained, the testicle will twist around its axis and obstruct its blood supply. This is extremely painful, so the dog will have a very tense abdomen, may vomit and will be very reluctant to move. The blood supply is severely reduced by the torsion and this causes tissue death.

Treatment Emergency surgical removal is invariably necessary.

DISEASES OF THE PROSTATE GLAND

Infection

Acute prostatitis is an uncommon condition but can be seen in dogs of any age. An affected dog is subdued, off his food, has a raised temperature, abdominal pain and is usually reluctant to move. He may strain to pass urine and any passed may contain traces of blood. His prostate will be enlarged and painful; this can be detected during a rectal examination by the vet, who may also be able to feel this enlarged gland by palpating the abdomen.

Treatment This infection usually responds readily to specific antibiotics, the choice of

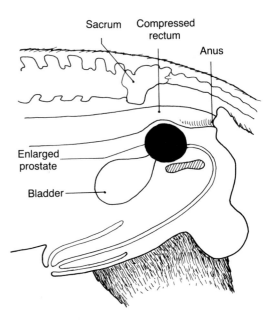

Fig 40 *An enlarged prostate can cause constipation or obstruction to urine flow*

which will depend on the result of a culture from the urine or any discharge from the penis.

Prostatic abscesses are much more serious and are usually seen in the older dog. The onset of symptoms is slower but the signs are similar to those of prostatitis. Prostatic abscesses are very difficult to treat as antibiotics often have little effect. Even surgical drainage of the abscess is difficult and gives poor results.

Prostatic Enlargement

This is a condition of the old dog in which the prostate slowly increases in size. This enlarged prostate presses upwards against the rectum in the pelvic canal and so may produce either faecal straining or constipation. The enlarged prostate can be felt on a rectal examination or demonstrated on an X-ray.

Treatment An enlarged prostate will reduce in size following large doses of a female hormone or, more permanently, following surgical castration. Initially, however, an affected dog may require an enema to empty the rectum and should then be fed low-bulk food such as fish and rice, until the prostate has reduced in size.

Prostatic Cysts

Very occasionally large, hard-walled cysts develop from the prostate. Symptoms are similar to those of an enlarged prostate and surgical removal may be necessary.

Tumours

The prostate is not a common site for tumour development. The initial symptoms caused by prostatic tumours resemble those of prostatic enlargement but there is little response to hormonal therapy. In the later stages, the tumour may damage the urethra causing urinary straining with usually blood in the urine.

Treatment Surgical removal of prostatic tumours is not usually successful so affected dogs are normally euthanased when the condition causes discomfort.

DISEASES OF THE PENIS AND PREPUCE

Most adult male dogs will have an intermittent thick, greenish discharge from the prepuce. This is completely normal.

Balanitis

This infection of the penis and prepuce is not very common. An affected dog shows an increase in this discharge which may become reddish, and the dog will lick his penis more frequently.

Treatment This consists of flushing the prepuce with an antiseptic or an antibiotic solution. Sometimes antibiotics are needed in tablet or injection form.

Cuts

Occasionally, the penis may be injured and, because of its vascular nature, even small cuts will bleed profusely.

Treatment It is usually necessary to suture these under a general anaesthetic using dissolving stitches.

Dog Pox

This is an uncommon viral infection which produces small blisters, or vesicles, on the penis, prepuce and around the anus. It causes a mild irritation only.

Treatment The disease will resolve spontaneously so treatment is unnecessary.

Transmissible Venereal Tumour

This tumour is more common in tropical climates and is only rarely seen in Great Britain. The tumour spreads from dog to bitch, and vice versa, during mating and produces haemorrhagic masses around the base of the penis.

Treatment Surgical removal is difficult and the tumours often regrow.

Prolapse of the Penis (Paraphimosis)

If the opening of the prepuce is particularly narrow, a dog may be unable to retract his penis following an erection. This is called paraphimosis.

Treatment Usually, the penis can be replaced by the use of petroleum jelly as a lubricant, but sometimes an anaesthetic is necessary. If this becomes a recurring problem, surgery is required to increase the size of the prepucial opening. This condition is dealt with more fully in Chapter 18 (*see* page 225).

CASTRATION

Castration is of value in the treatment of some dog behavioural problems but will be successful only where the behaviour is, to some degree, influenced by the male hormones. Excessive sexual activity, such as mounting cushions or other dogs, and territorial urination may be eliminated by castration but many young dogs pass through this phase and then grow out of it. Certain types of aggression may be reduced by castration, as may the desire to escape and wander. Results, however, vary. Problems such as over-excitability and constant barking will not be affected. Behavioural problems and their treatment are discussed in greater detail in Chapter 17.

Castrated dogs put on weight more easily and require less food. However, if their diet is controlled and exercise maintained, they will remain as slim and athletic as entire dogs, although most show a slight change of shape and become more thickset at the waist.

Vasectomy

Where infertility is required but a change of behaviour is not, and where the desire to mate is not a disadvantage, it is possible for the vet to perform a vasectomy.

THE FEMALE DOG (BITCH) NORMAL STRUCTURE AND FUNCTION

The function of the female reproductive system is the production of eggs, the stimulation of the bitch to mate with the male, the conception and development of foetal puppies in the uterus and the rearing of these puppies until weaning. The reproductive system consists of paired ovaries, a Y-shaped uterus leading through the cervix to the vagina. In addition, the five paired mammary glands produce milk to rear the young.

The ovaries are small, glandular structures situated one behind each kidney in a little pouch called the ovarian bursa, which is connected to the uterus by a short fine tube, the Fallopian tube. Eggs are produced in the ovary and when released, pass across the bursa and enter the uterus along these Fallopian tubes. The ovaries also produce hormones which are released into the bloodstream to prepare the uterus for pregnancy and also help to maintain pregnancy. The horns of the uterus in the bitch are long and narrow and they join together to form a short uterine body which is normally sealed from the vagina by the muscular cervix. The cervix relaxes during each heat period to allow the introduction of sperm, and also during parturition (labour) so the foetuses can be expelled. The vagina connects the cervix to the vestibule which is the common opening for the reproductive and urinary systems. The vulva is the external visible entrance to the vestibule. (*See* Fig 38b.)

The five pairs of mammary glands are situated on the under-side of the chest and belly as a continuous strip from the axilla to the groin. Mammary development occurs after a heat period, during a false pregnancy or during a true pregnancy. The mammary glands reach maximum size two to three weeks after parturition.

THE NORMAL OESTROUS CYCLE OR HEAT PERIOD

A bitch will normally come on heat every six months although in some it can be every nine to twelve months. This heat period is divided into pro-oestrus, oestrus, metoestrus and anoestrus. Pro-oestrus and oestrus are referred to as the heat.

In pro-oestrus the vulva starts to swell and most bitches show a watery haemorrhagic discharge. The bitch will not accept the dog during this period which lasts about nine days.

Oestrus follows on and lasts again about nine days. During this period the bitch is receptive to the dog. The haemorrhagic discharge is usually less profuse but more tacky. Ovulation occurs early in oestrus and so the best time for mating is between the tenth and thirteenth day after the first signs of heat are noticed.

Metoestrus follows the oestrus in an unmated bitch. It is during this period that

false pregnancies develop because the hormone levels are similar to those of the pregnant bitch. This period can last up to ninety days.

Anoestrus is the period of inactivity in the bitch's reproductive cycle, when everything returns to normal before the next heat.

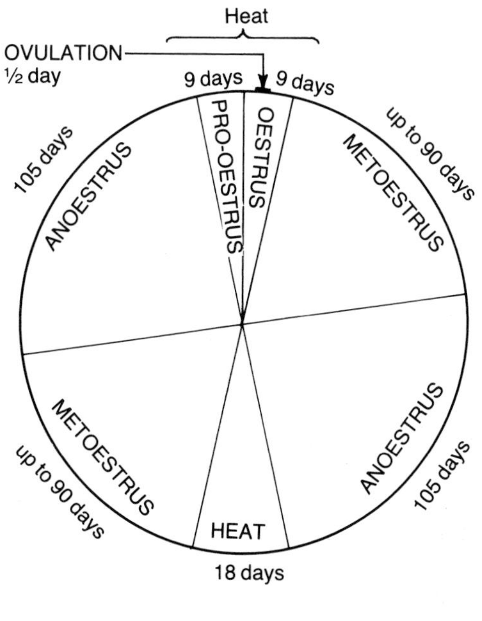

DISEASES OF THE OVARIES

Cystic Ovaries

During the heat period the ovary produces follicles which contain the egg and produce hormones. Sometimes, these follicles are produced at the wrong time so the bitch may have prolonged or irregular heat periods which may recur after a short interval. During these abnormal periods the follicles do not rupture but form a cyst and as the eggs are not released, the bitch is often sterile. Very rarely these cystic ovaries can cause abdominal discomfort.

Treatment Hormonal treatment is often unrewarding and a surgical operation to remove the ovaries and uterus, called an ovarohysterectomy or spay operation, is the treatment preferred.

Ovarian Tumours

These tumours are very rare but are usually highly malignant. There may be some evidence of hormonal change, such as vulval swelling and bleeding, but signs of disease are usually related to the organs to which the tumour has spread, such as the kidney or liver. These tumours are almost always inoperable.

Fig 41 Annual breeding cycle of the bitch (all times are approximate)

187

DISEASES OF THE UTERUS

Metritis

Metritis is an inflammation of the uterus and is caused by an infection which gains entry when the cervix is open during oestrus or after whelping. The condition is more common in young dogs. A reddish discharge is seen which continues longer than that of a normal heat period. The bitch repeatedly licks at her vulva and she may be lethargic.

Treatment Metritis readily responds to antibiotic therapy.

Pyometritis (Pyometra)

This is a very common and serious disease of the old, entire (not spayed) bitch, although bitches which have had puppies seem less likely to develop pyometra. Infection can gain entry into the uterus as before but, in many cases of pyometra, no infective agent can be found. There is a slow buildup of pus and an affected uterus can approach the normal full-term pregnant size. The bitch slowly becomes poisoned by the release of toxins from the pus into her bloodstream.

Symptoms The symptoms normally become apparent shortly after a heat period. Initially, there will be abdominal distension, loss of appetite and an excess thirst due to the toxicity and kidney damage. If untreated, vomiting often occurs and the bitch will appear very ill, dull and may have a purulent conjunctivitis of her eyes.

Further symptoms shown depend on whether the pyometra is 'open' or 'closed'. In an open pyometra, the cervix relaxes and pus can drain through the vulva. Therefore, the diagnosis of an open pyometra is more straightforward and, because pus is released, the bitch is usually less ill than one with a closed pyometra where there is no leakage of pus. This latter condition can be difficult to diagnose as many other problems of the old bitch will produce similar symptoms. However, the enlarged uterus can usually be seen on an X-ray, or detected by the vet on abdominal palpation. Blood tests can confirm the diagnosis but, as the condition is often an emergency, an exploratory operation is usually performed.

Treatment Once a diagnosis has been made, treatment is normally instigated immediately. Hormonal treatment for releasing the pus from the uterus is available, but it is not always reliable and not without risks. The most effective treatment, in our opinion, is an ovarohysterectomy. An affected bitch can be very ill and will usually require intravenous fluid therapy to counteract the shock and dehydration that accompany this condition. Antibiotic cover is normally given following the operation.

DISEASES OF THE VAGINA

Juvenile Vaginitis

This is described in Chapter 4 (*see* page 56).

Adult Vaginitis

This disease is often associated with damage at mating, foreign bodies, and polyps or tumours of the vagina. It can be a primary infection in kennels where outbreaks may occur due to a bacterium, *Beta haemolytic streptococcus* which can cause infertility. The symptoms include a discharge which causes the bitch to lick the vulva excessively.

Treatment The removal of foreign bodies or tumours is essential, and antibiotic treatment after sensitivity testing of the discharge.

Vaginal Hyperplasia

During a heat period, the lining of the vagina may swell up to produce a balloon-like mass which appears at the vulva. After the heat period has finished, the swelling regresses. This is an uncommon condition seen mainly in the Boxer, and will cause problems with mating. However, if your vet feels it is necessary, the affected tissue can be removed surgically.

Tumours

The vagina is an uncommon site for malignant tumour growth, but benign, often multiple, polyps are seen. The symptoms which can resemble those of vaginitis, are those of a watery reddish discharge and vulval irritation. Occasionally, the first sign is the tumour appearing at the vulva.

Treatment Surgical removal is the preferred treatment.

Dog Pox

Dog pox is similar to the disease in the male dog, but the pox lesions appear in the vagina. These may cause a mild irritation, causing the bitch to lick herself repeatedly. There is no treatment available, but the disease usually resolves spontaneously.

Transmissible Venereal Tumour

This is also similar to the disease in the male dog, but the haemorrhagic lesions are present in the vagina. Surgery is complicated, but a few cases will regress spontaneously.

DISEASES OF THE MAMMARY GLANDS

Mastitis

Infection of the mammary glands and the inflammation it causes is called mastitis. It is extremely rare in spayed bitches, but is seen more often in lactating bitches, where the infection can enter one or more glands following pregnancy or even a false pregnancy. The affected glands become swollen and hard, and the bitch may have a raised temperature and be reluctant to feed the puppies because the condition is painful. Any milk produced will become blood tinged or discoloured.

Treatment This type of mastitis responds readily to antibiotic therapy, provided treatment is instigated early in the course of the disease.

Very occasionally, infection will enter an inactive gland to produce a severe infection. The affected gland becomes very swollen and painful, the bitch develops a high temperature, becomes lethargic and refuses to eat.

Treatment Antibiotic treatment will reduce the swelling and lower the temperature, but the gland is usually so damaged that surgical removal is necessary. Mild chronic infection can occur and this causes small hard nodules scattered throughout the glands. These rarely cause problems, but they can be difficult to differentiate from early tumour formation on clinical signs alone. A biopsy will, however, identify the problem.

Tumours

Mammary tumours are very common in the older entire bitch, less common if the bitch was spayed at an early age and extremely rare in a bitch spayed before her first heat. Any breast can be affected, but tumours seem to occur more frequently in the rear glands. Most tumours are benign, but where malignant they can grow very rapidly and spread to other organs. If a tumour is left untreated, it increases in size and causes the skin to overstretch and ulcerate, producing a septic, sore, discharging area which does not respond to medical treatment.

Treatment   Early surgical removal of any lump discovered in the mammary glands is advisable because of the danger of malignancy. In the case of multiple or extensive tumours, it will be necessary to remove several glands and, in some cases, all the mammary tissue. This latter operation, known as a mammary strip, is very well tolerated by the bitch and an ideal way to remove multiple tumours.

FALSE PREGNANCY

A false or pseudo-pregnancy occurs in most bitches and can be regarded as a normal occurrence. The symptoms appear about eight to twelve weeks after oestrus at the stage when the bitch would be lactating had she been pregnant. This also occurs in wolf and wild dog packs and is useful as false pregnant bitches can help in the suckling of young. We have helped orphaned puppies in this way by locating a lactating false pregnant bitch.

Symptoms   The severity of the symptoms can be very variable, and include poor appetite, lethargy, milk production, nest building, aggressiveness and attachment to a substitute puppy – often a squeaky toy. Once a bitch has had a false pregnancy, she is likely to have one after each heat period.

Treatment   A mild false pregnancy does not require any treatment, but if the bitch is adversely affected, it can be suppressed with hormone therapy. False pregnancies can be prevented by suppressing oestrus with a hormone injection, or tablets. Once the ovaries are removed surgically by a spay operation, the bitch will have no more false pregnancies.

BIRTH CONTROL

Hormone Therapy

Several hormone preparations, both in tablet or injection form, are available to prevent or postpone the bitch's heat period. The main value of these is to prevent an occasional heat where, for instance, it might occur during a holiday or an important show. There are, however, reliable preparations that may be prescribed by your vet on a regular basis for the permanent or semi-permanent postponement of heats.

In the vast majority of cases, once the use of these preparations ceases, the ovaries begin to function normally again. Very occasionally, however, irregular heat periods may ensue.

Spaying

A spay operation (ovarohysterectomy) is an operation to remove the uterus and ovaries, and it is usually performed to prevent the problems associated with oestrus and false or unwanted pregnancies. Spaying also has other beneficial effects as it prevents pyometra and, if performed early in life, greatly reduces the chance of the bitch suffering from mammary tumours, mastitis and diabetes mellitus. Spaying also prevents the problems associated with the bitch wandering while on heat, such as road traffic accidents. Also, the gathering of male dogs around the bitch's home while she is on heat can be a major nuisance.

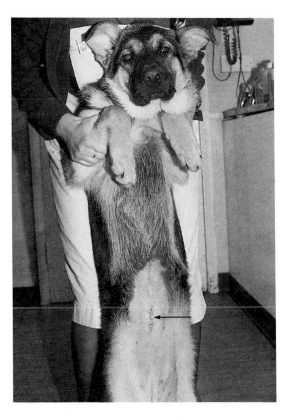

Six-month-old German Shepherd Dog puppy, four hours after her spay.

There are some potential minor disadvantages to spaying. The coat of the feathered breeds, such as the Spaniels, Retrievers and Afghan Hound, may occasionally become woolly, but this does not affect the general health of the bitch. A few spayed bitches, especially those of the giant breeds, may suffer from urinary incontinence later in life, but this problem is usually controlled with a short course of replacement hormones. A spayed bitch is more likely to become overweight as her appetite may increase, but this is easily controlled by attention to diet and exercise.

16 Breeding and Associated Problems

MATING

The bitch comes into heat on average twice a year and only during this period will she mate. Each heat consists of a pro-oestrus period of seven to ten days, during which the males become interested but the bitch will not allow mating, followed by oestrus proper, lasting for a further seven to ten days, when she will allow mating. At this stage the vulva is enlarged and engorged and ready to accept the penis of the male.

She will signal her acceptance of the male by standing still with her tail slightly raised and turned to one side to expose the vulva. Often, she will orientate herself so that her vulva is towards the male and then back up to him. The male, usually after a little investigation to ensure she is receptive, mounts the bitch from the rear and inserts his penis into the bitch's vagina. The penis now erect, is enlarged even further by the swelling of glands at the base, and is locked into position inside the female. This produces the so called 'tie' and, after a minute or so of copulation, the male, with his penis still inside the bitch's vagina, lifts one hind leg over her back and places it on the ground. The two dogs stand back to back for up to twenty minutes until the penis subsides and they can separate. This tie ensures that the maximum amount of semen reaches the uterus and increases the chances of fertilization. A tie, although preferable, is not essential and pregnancies frequently result from 'slip services' where ejaculation occurs without a tie.

It is advisable to mate the two dogs at least twice on successive days, around the eleventh day of heat, if possible. However, a greater success rate is achieved if the dogs are allowed to run together for a while on each of several successive days.

MISMATING (MISALLIANCE)

If an unwanted mating has, or is thought to have, occurred and a pregnancy is not wanted, it is possible for the vet to give an injection of an oestrogen hormone to prevent implantation of the fertilised eggs in the uterus. This must be given within three days of the mating.

PROBLEMS AT MATING

If the bitch fails to stand for the male, you should check that the stage of heat is correct. Normally this would be about the tenth to twelfth day, but some breeds, for example the Bull Terrier, ovulate very late, up to the nineteenth day of oestrus. Also, individuals within a breed vary and may be ready to mate earlier or later than expected. If in doubt, your vet can take vaginal smears to ascertain whether she is at the correct stage to mate. This is called vaginal cytology.

Vaginal Cytology

As the timing of ovulation varies from bitch to bitch, the ideal time to mate her varies also. Ovulation occurs early in oestrus itself

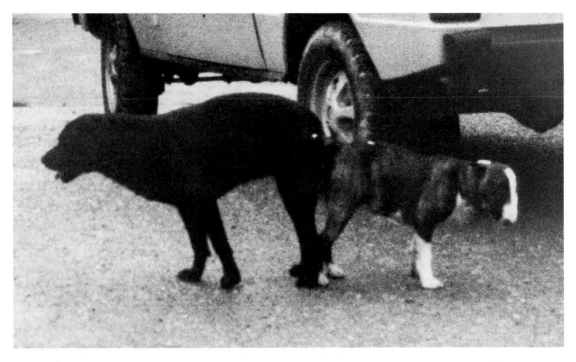

The 'tie' during a mis-mating.

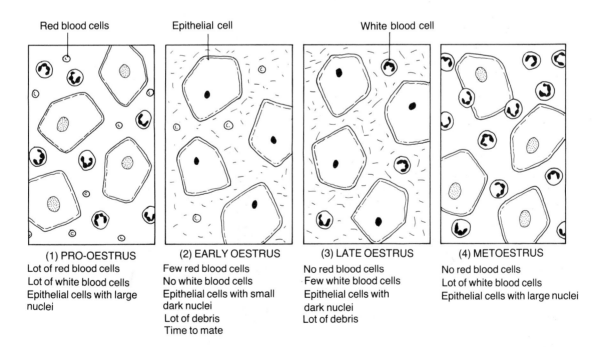

(1) PRO-OESTRUS
Lot of red blood cells
Lot of white blood cells
Epithelial cells with large
nuclei

(2) EARLY OESTRUS
Few red blood cells
No white blood cells
Epithelial cells with small
dark nuclei
Lot of debris
Time to mate

(3) LATE OESTRUS
No red blood cells
Few white blood cells
Epithelial cells with
dark nuclei
Lot of debris

(4) METOESTRUS
No red blood cells
Lot of white blood cells
Epithelial cells with large nuclei

Fig 42 Vaginal cytology (cells seen in the vagina at various stages of the heat cycle)

193

so a test to determine when oestrus started will indicate the ideal time to mate. At the start of oestrus, the vaginal discharge contains many dead epithelial lining cells, and a lot of debris. By now there are no red blood cells present and as yet no white blood cells. Thus the microscopic examination of a vaginal swab taken daily by the vet will indicate when oestrus starts and therefore when to mate.

MALE INFERTILITY

Infertility can be caused by sterility, lack of libido or both. Libido is the desire to mate and some male dogs refuse to mate for various reasons. Dogs become sexually mature at different ages and an immature dog, who is under two years of age, may merely be reluctant to mate, as may an old dog, because libido also decreases with old age. Low levels of male hormones, due to retained or damaged testicles, will also reduce sexual appetite. There may be other, more obvious causes, however. For instance, the dog may be reluctant to mate because of pain in his sex organs, or even in his spine, hips or hind legs.

The investigation of poor libido firstly requires the elimination of any concurrent disease or behaviour problem. If none is present, hormone therapy may be tried to raise the male hormone levels.

Sterility is the inability to reproduce and, in the male dog, is usually caused by a defective or nil sperm count. A sample of semen can be examined under the microscope to ascertain the total sperm count and to assess whether the sperms are normal or deformed. Diseases of the testicles and prostate may also produce sterility. If there is no obvious disease of the male reproductive tract, hormone therapy may improve the dog's fertility.

FEMALE INFERTILITY

Failure to Mate

If the bitch fails to develop a full heat period, she may fail to mate or the owner may miss the signs and not take the bitch to be mated. A 'silent' heat can be caused by a low hormone level, or by damage to the ovaries. However, another reason for failure may be that the bitch is physically unable to mate due to such conditions as back or hip pain, vaginal hyperplasia, or tumours, strictures, or excessive narrowing of the vagina. Some bitches can be very temperamental and refuse to mate with a particular dog or in strange surroundings.

A stricture within the vagina may lead to a failure of mating. If the bitch shows signs of discomfort and moves away, consult your vet who will give her a physical examination.

Failure to Conceive

Conception requires the release of eggs into the uterus and fertilisation of these by sperm. As sperm can survive only for up to two days in the female genital tract, the timing of mating is very important but it is not always easy to predict exactly when the eggs will be released. Ovulation usually occurs on the tenth to twelfth day of heat but multiple matings over a few days are advisable to increase the chance of fertilisation. Failure of egg release or the inability of the egg to enter the uterus, due to damage to the ovarian bursa or Fallopian tube, will cause infertility.

After the egg is fertilised it becomes embedded (implanted) in the uterine wall. Here a placenta forms from which the growing foetus gains its nutrients through the umbilical cord. Sometimes the fertilised egg may fail to implant, either due to infection of the uterus or failure of the hormone responsible for implantation.

If the bitch fails to conceive, try again at the next heat and consider a different male. There may be nothing wrong individually with either the dog or bitch but together they may be incompatible. If the male, despite mating normally, repeatedly fails to father a litter, he may be infertile.

PREGNANCY

In the bitch the gestation period, or length of pregnancy, is normally sixty-three days, although variations of up to seven days can occur. For the first three weeks, there is little noticeable change in either the behaviour or the appearance of the bitch. She may, however, be quieter than normal and look a little plump. Some development of the breasts occurs at this stage and the teats may begin to enlarge.

At about three and a half to four and a half weeks after mating, your vet may be able to tell you if she is pregnant by gently feeling her abdomen. In the average pregnant bitch, the enlargement of the uterus around each developing puppy may be felt as a swelling the size of a ping-pong ball. Later, each swelling becomes larger and softer and difficult to distinguish from bowel, until about the seventh week when the puppies themselves are substantial enough to be detected by palpation. There is now a blood test which can detect pregnancy from about three and a half weeks. Ultrasound scanning, which is available in a very few veterinary practices, will confirm pregnancy at about the same stage.

From about the sixth week of pregnancy, the bitch begins to show a more obvious increase in size of the abdomen and the teats and mammary glands begin to enlarge. She will usually become a little more sedate but her appetite remains good. At this stage, food intake should be increased and it is advisable to include a balanced vitamin and mineral supplement in her diet. There are several useful products available in either tablet or powder form, which can be obtained from your vet.

About a week before she is due to give birth (whelp), milk may start to ooze from the teats, and the bitch will begin to slow down. The onset of first-stage labour is signalled by a change in behaviour of the bitch, and a thermometer will show that her temperature has dropped considerably. It will drop from 38.5°C (101.5°F) to as low as 36°C (97°F). This is a definite sign of impending birth.

PROBLEMS DURING PREGNANCY

Abortion

Loss of the foetus can occur after implantation. If the loss occurs early in pregancy, the small foetuses are simply reabsorbed through the uterine wall, whereas later in pregnancy the foetuses will be aborted. Reabsorption or abortion can occur from foetal overcrowding, hormonal failure or an infection which may either be localised to the uterus or generalised. An ill bitch may be unable to support a pregnancy.

Abortion is uncommon, but in our experience once a miscarriage has started to occur, there is little that can be done to halt it. However, occasionally an injection of progesterone, the hormone responsible for maintaining pregnancy, will enable the bitch to hold on to her puppies. If the abortion continues, veterinary supervision is essential to ensure all is well.

BIRTH (PARTURITION, LABOUR OR WHELPING)

It is essential that a whelping box, or something similar, has been prepared for the bitch to whelp in. There will be a lot of fluid discharge, usually green, during the birth and it is a good idea to pad the box with several layers of newspaper which can gradually be removed, as they become soiled. It is easier to remove soiled newspaper than to add fresh. A typical whelping box is shown in Fig 43 below. The dimensions will vary according to the breed but a general rule is that the bitch should be able to stretch out in either direction with the safety bar in place. An infra-red heat source directly over the whelping area is vital to prevent the puppies developing hypothermia.

First-Stage Labour

First-stage labour is characterised by a gradually developing restlessness on the part of the bitch. The bitch appears uneasy, and usually indulges in bed-making. She may tear up newspaper or scatter blankets around. This stage occurs as the cervix is widening to allow passage of the puppies and as the first puppy is being moved towards the cervix. It can last for up to twenty-four hours but it is usually much shorter. Towards the end of the period contractions begin to develop.

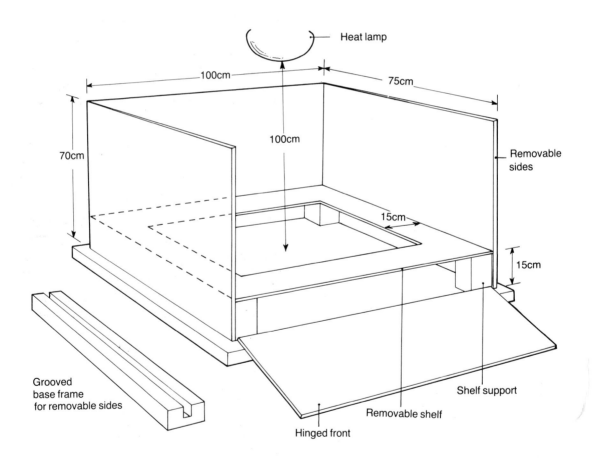

Fig 43 Whelping box for a medium-sized bitch

Second-Stage Labour

Initially, the contractions are several minutes apart but they gradually increase in frequency until the bitch's abdomen is contracting several times each minute. This is the beginning of second-stage labour which is the stage during which the puppies are born. The first sign is a water bag appearing at the vulva. A puppy is usually born within twenty minutes of the onset of regular rhythmical contractions, but this can take up to two hours in a normal whelping. Thereafter, the interval between puppies varies enormously. We have known bitches rest for twelve hours after delivering the puppies from one horn of the uterus before giving birth normally to the remaining ones. However, an interval of ten to sixty minutes between each puppy is more usual.

Each puppy is contained in a fluid-filled membrane bag in the uterus and has his own placenta attached to the uterine lining. He may be born enclosed in the bag or this may have ruptured during birth. By licking the puppy immediately after birth, the bitch will usually rupture the bag and revive him, and he will very shortly begin to cry as he fills his lungs for the first time. If the bitch ignores the puppy or seems confused, the owner must gently but firmly tear the bag from around the puppy, hold him in a towel, wipe out the mouth and vigorously rub the puppy within the towel to stimulate breathing. If the placenta or afterbirth is attached to the puppy, the umbilical cord should be tied with cotton about one and a half inches from the puppy and carefully cut with scissors on the placenta side of the knot. The puppy should then be placed gently in the whelping box and on to a teat when he will normally begin suckling.

Third-Stage Labour

The placenta is usually passed immediately after the puppy and is still attached to him by the umbilical cord. Very often, however, the placenta becomes detached as the umbilical cord ruptures due to the vigour of birth, and it remains inside the uterus. This is perfectly normal and should not be a worry to the owner. Retained placentae will slowly disintegrate and be expelled from the uterus as a darkish discharge over the next few weeks. If the placenta is expelled, it will usually be eaten by the bitch and this should be encouraged.

The bitch will pay nominal attention to each puppy as he is born but will not normally be very interested in the litter until whelping is over. Then a change in attitude is usually obvious. The bitch will brighten up, clean herself thoroughly and begin to look after the puppies in earnest.

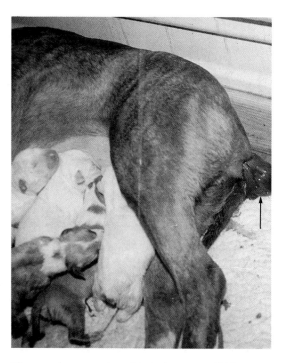

The water bag appearing with the last puppy of this Bull Terrier litter.

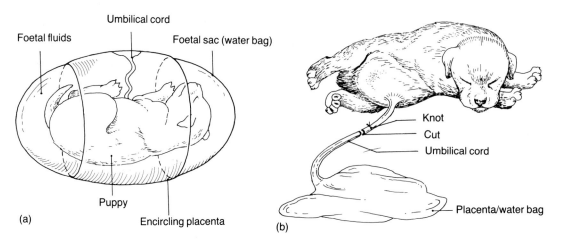

Fig 44 (a) Foetus just before birth
(b) New-born puppy showing where to cut the umbilical cord

PROBLEMS AT WHELPING

Primary Inertia

This is a condition whereby the bitch simply fails to start second-stage labour. She has no contractions at all, despite showing all the signs of first-stage labour including a dilated cervix and temperature fall. If whelping does not follow within twenty-four hours of the onset of first-stage labour, if the bitch is more than one day overdue or if a vaginal discharge is noticed, she should be examined by a vet in case inertia is present.

Treatment An injection of a hormone, oxytocin, may stimulate contractions and your vet may decide to use this if the cervix is opening.

A Caesarean section may be the course of action decided on. This is an operation during which the puppies are removed surgically and revived in the operating theatre. This operation is well tolerated by bitch and puppies alike. Within twenty-four hours the bitch is usually alert and is suckling her puppies well. Sometimes, due to foetal death for instance, all is not well and the vet may have to prescribe hormones to cause reabsorption of the milk in the absence of any puppies.

Secondary Inertia

This usually follows a prolonged unproductive labour where due to an obstruction, called dystocia, birth cannot take place and the bitch becomes exhausted. This obstruction can be caused by uterine or other maternal factors (maternal dystocia), or an abnormally formed or positioned foetus (foetal dystocia). A dystocia must be suspected where the bitch has been contracting unproductively for over two hours.

Maternal Dystocia

There are three main causes:

Pelvic Fracture

This causes a narrowing of the birth canal and is invariably the result of a previous road accident. A bitch who suffers a pelvic fracture should be spayed to eliminate the possibility of pregnancy.

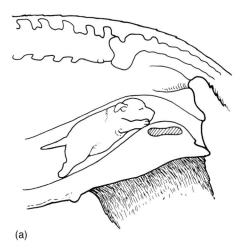

(a)

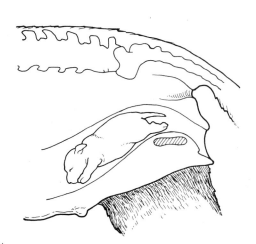

(c)

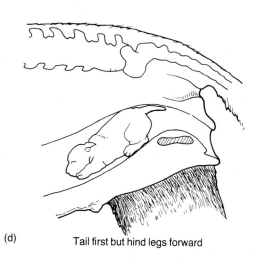

(b)   Head forward but front legs back

(d)   Tail first but hind legs forward

Fig 45 Puppy positions at whelping
    (a) Normal anterior presentation
    (b) Abnormal, head forward but not legs

    (c) Normal posterior presentation
    (d) Abnormal, breech presentation

Uterine Twist (Torsion)

This usually occurs in the bitch who is heavily pregnant with a large number of puppies present in the uterus. It is thought to be due to rotation of this heavy organ within the abdomen in response to an awkward movement of the bitch.

Treatment Both conditions necessitate a Caesarean section to preserve the life of the bitch and puppies.

Rupture of the Uterus

This can occur spontaneously and be due to trauma or follow a twist of the uterus. The bitch will show signs of pain or profound depression.

Treatment A Caesarean section is necessary and usually also involves a hysterectomy due to severe damage to the uterus.

Foetal Dystocia

Over-Large Puppy

This can be a genuine, oversized puppy particularly in a single puppy litter. The puppy may, on the other hand, be relatively oversized due to a small birth canal. Invariably the first puppy to be born causes the problem and if successfully delivered, the rest usually follow.

Malpresentation

Puppies are born either head and forelegs first (anterior presentation) or tail and back legs first (posterior presentation). Both are normal and easily delivered. Any variations on this can cause foetal dystocia. Two common examples are:

Breech presentation This is where the tail is presenting first but the hind legs are tucked up under the puppy's abdomen as if it were in a sitting position. This greatly enlarges the buttocks of the puppy and causes an obstruction.

Treatment If possible, the puppy should be gently pushed back a little with a finger, which may then be able to hook one hind leg back at a time to line up with the tail, enabling delivery of the puppy. Copious lubrication is essential.

Head first with forelegs pointing backwards If the puppy is presented in this position delivery is prevented because the shoulders are grossly enlarged.

Treatment Hook the legs forward gently with a finger one at a time to enable delivery to take place.

Congenital Abnormalities

Congenital abnormalities can result in misformed puppies which may be difficult or impossible for the bitch to deliver. These are diagnosed usually only on Caesarean section. Most puppies do not survive and, indeed, if a severe abnormality exists, euthanasia at birth may be the kindest course of action.

POST-NATAL PROBLEMS IN THE BITCH

Failure of Milk

Sometimes the bitch fails to produce milk and the mammary glands dry up. The puppies fail to thrive and cry continuously. It is essential to supplement feeding with a foster feeding bottle and synthetic milk, obtainable from your vet or local pet shop.

Vaginal Discharge

A greenish brown discharge is normal for the first few days after whelping and may continue for several weeks. Provided the bitch is otherwise well there should be no cause for worry.

Post-Whelping Metritis

This usually occurs after a prolonged whelping, or one where a dystocia occurred, and may be associated with the retention of a placenta or foetal membranes. An affected bitch will appear very ill within about twenty-four hours of whelping and she will have a copious, foul smelling brown discharge from her vulva. Her temperature will usually be raised to 40°C (104°F).

Treatment An antibiotic is administered in high doses or occasionally an ovarohysterectomy operation is required. Despite treatment, some bitches with this condition will die. This type of metritis is often associated with the development of mastitis.

Mastitis

This can occur in over-engorged mammary glands. Check daily that no breasts are sore, very hard or hot.

Treatment Mastitis must be treated immediately with an antibiotic and puppies should be removed and hand-reared while the bitch is undergoing treatment.

Behavioural Change

The bitch may become very protective over her puppies, even to the extent of being aggressive with her owner. If this develops it is wise to leave bitch and puppies alone to start with, provided the puppies are checked from time to time in the bitch's absence. After a few days as the situation becomes more familiar to the bitch, her worries will subside and she will become trusting again. If handling is necessary, for instance to supplement the puppies, a muzzle may be necessary.

Aggression to Puppies

This can occur in the first few days and the bitch must be muzzled or the puppies separated. Usually this is fright, confusion or displaced excessive cleaning. Once they have been forcibly held on to her to be suckled for a while, she will normally accept them.

Eclampsia (Milk Fever)

This is a terrifying condition for the owner and can be fatal for the bitch. The blood calcium level of the bitch becomes too low,

due to the puppies' demands for her milk, and she begins to show nervous symptoms. To start with she may just look a little odd by twitching or shivering and appearing unsteady. This rapidly progresses to obvious staggering, a wide-eyed frightened expression and convulsions. It is essential that the vet is contacted immediately as an injection of calcium, usually directly into a vein, is essential to save the life of the bitch. The response is dramatic and, within a few minutes, she is walking normally again.

However, once the blood calcium has been this low, the puppies should be weaned from her to ensure the eclampsia does not recur. The time of onset varies but it is usually seen when the puppies are about three weeks old and making maximum demands on her.

It may be possible to prevent eclampsia by ensuring an adequate calcium intake during pregnancy and lactation. But, other factors are involved as eclampsia can still occur despite increased calcium levels. It is usually seen in small bitches with large litters, so supplementing the puppies' diet to relieve the load on the dam would also seem to be a logical approach to prevention.

POST-NATAL PROBLEMS OF THE PUPPIES

Days One and Two

Check all the puppies to ensure there are no obvious congenital abnormalities present. If in doubt the vet should be asked to attend. You should check for:

Hare lip
Cleft palate
Atresia ani (absence of an anus) We have seen this on occasions. Sometimes, if the defect is slight, a new anus can be constructed but if a large segment of the colon is missing, euthanasia is essential.

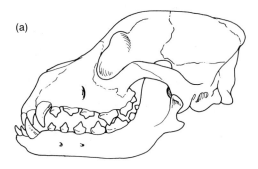

Fig 46 (a) Undershot jaw (b) Overshot jaw

Undershot/overshot jaws Exaggerated examples may be detected at this stage.

Any disruption during development of the foetus can lead to congenital abnormalities of a variety of types. Therefore, defects in the limbs, head, or spine can all be seen, but are uncommon.

Ensure the puppies all suckle the bitch on the first day. This is important as her first milk (colostrum) is rich in antibodies and is only produced for a day or two. The puppies can also only absorb these maternal antibodies for two days at the most. It is essential, therefore, they receive a good supply at this stage to enable them to withstand infections during their first six to twelve weeks of life. They will obtain antibodies to most diseases to which their mother is immune.

The puppies must have enough to drink. A quiet litter is usually a happy, well-fed litter. If any puppies are weaker, it may be necessary to supplement them with synthetic bitch's milk using a foster feeder bottle.

Days Three to Five

Dew Claws

Unless your breed requires hind dew claws for showing, for example the Pyrenean Mountain Dog, it is wise to ask your vet to remove them at this stage as they will become ungainly and curved like a hook if left. They will then be likely to catch in the undergrowth when the dog is fully grown resulting in a painful injury. It may be worth enquiring whether the front dew claws should also be removed although these become injured less often.

Tail Docking

Dogs need their tails for various reasons but mainly to assist them in communication. Tail docking is of no benefit to the puppy and is performed solely for fashion. In years to come, we expect to look back on this practice and wonder why it was ever carried out.

If you consider it necessary to dock a puppy's tail, it must be done at this age. A number of breeds have by tradition had their tails docked (Boxer, Poodle, Corgi, Dobermann, Yorkshire Terrier, to name but a few) and this has been essential for success at showing. However, even as this book goes to print, opinions seem to be changing. The Kennel Club have recently changed all the breed standards to make docking optional for showing. A proposed new European convention may even outlaw docking of dogs' tails to bring it in line with the docking of horses' tails and cropping of dogs' ears, neither of which are carried out in Great Britain now.

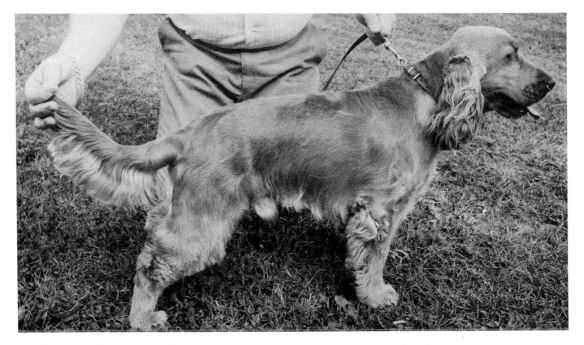

A golden Cocker Spaniel with a tail.

Days Five to Fourteen

The eyes open at ten to fourteen days and at this stage any abnormality is noticed. Occasionally, an eye may be absent (anophthalmia) or much smaller than normal (microphthalmia). These are both congenital abnormalities.

At fourteen days, you should consult your vet about the treatment of roundworm infestation – a parasite of the bowel.

Fading Puppy Syndrome

As the name implies, puppies begin to fade and die for no apparent reason. Indeed, the problem is often multifactoral, meaning there are several possible causes. It is essential that the vet is consulted, and helpful if you can provide him with the dead puppy on which he can perform a post-mortem examination to reach a diagnosis. The cause may be hypothermia, infection, lack of food, or colostrum, trauma from the bitch, roundworms or any stress.

Two to Three Weeks

The puppies become more mobile after the eyes open, and at three weeks they are fairly lively and capable of wandering out of the whelping area and around the room. This is a useful period to begin socialising with them.

Three to Six Weeks

At three weeks weaning can begin. The puppies should be taught to lap a specially formulated milk substitute (obtainable from your vet) or diluted or skimmed cow's milk to start with. Within a few days, they can be fed with a small amount of porridge-style cereals or even a little boiled, mashed fish or finely minced chicken. It is important to feed them several times a day but at this stage, they will still be suckling the bitch as well.

By four weeks they should have progressed to four or five small meals a day, such as fresh meat or tinned puppy food mixed with

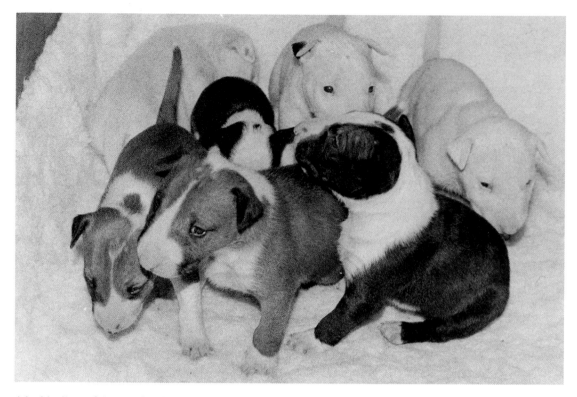

A healthy litter of three-week-old Bull Terrier puppies.

a little soaked breakfast cereal or puppy cereal. A balanced vitamin and mineral supplement should be added daily or given in the form of a tasty tablet. These can be obtained from your veterinary surgeon.

WORMING

The puppies should be wormed at two weeks of age and thereafter at intervals of two weeks, up to the age of three months, using a safe but effective veterinary wormer. Thereafter, worming should be carried out at four, five and six months of age and then two to four times a year for the rest of their lives.

Puppies still in the uterus can become infected with roundworm larvae through the placenta. This can be minimised by giving a larvicidal wormer, obtainable from your vet, to the bitch during pregnancy and lactation. Your vet should be consulted for details of dosage and timing. In addition, the bitch should be dosed each time the puppies are wormed in an attempt to prevent the buildup of a roundworm burden within the litter and its environment. Worming is discussed in greater detail in Chapter 6 (*see* pages 87–90).

THE NEW HOME

The best age for the puppy to adapt to a new family is between six and ten weeks of age. This, therefore, is the age at which you should aim to sell them. Remember the puppy will make a better pet if you and your family have been playing with him gently and handling him.

Before parting with a puppy you should:

1 Interview the prospective purchasers to ensure that they will give the puppy a caring home and that he will suit their life style.

2 Make sure that the puppy is fit and well.

3 Prepare a diet sheet to give to the new owners.

4 Inform them about the worming programme carried out so far and when the next worming is due.

5 Hand out the vaccination certificate if the first vaccination has been given.

6 Prepare the pedigree form, if applicable.

7 Take out a temporary pet health insurance policy on the puppy. This lasts for six weeks and the new owner should be advised to continue it. It relieves you of the worry of any unforeseen illness or problem in the first few weeks after purchase. It is not expensive and your vet will give you details.

17 Behavioural Problems

Most owners regard their dog as one of the family and, therefore, the dog has to fit into family life. Thus, he must be hygienic and not urinate or defaecate indoors, he must not be aggressive to members of the family, people in general or other animals, he must not rip the home to pieces, he must be obedient to his owners and he must be sociable. Any behaviour which deviates from the so-called normal can be classed as a behavioural problem and, increasingly, veterinary surgeons are being consulted on such problems by worried owners.

CAUSES OF BEHAVIOURAL PROBLEMS

Abnormal behaviour can be attributed to:

1 Incorrect training during puppyhood. This includes lack of training whereby the puppy is 'trained' to realise he can do as he likes because no attempt is made to correct him. We strongly recommend inexperienced owners to attend local obedience classes with their puppy from about four months of age onwards, until the basic training is completed. *It is essential that owners understand that they need to be the pack leaders.*
2 Inherited behavioural problems. Certain strains of some breeds of dog have a high incidence of behavioural problems which have a hereditary component.
3 Normal behaviour patterns in the dog family (e.g. wolf, fox) which are unacceptable in the family dog. An example of this is territorial urinating.
4 Vices which develop in dogs who are not allowed to indulge in normal behaviour patterns. For example, a male dog who is never allowed to mate may well attempt to mount substitutes such as children or cushions.

By understanding the reasons for the dog's bad behaviour and appreciating what must be done to correct it and why, it is possible to eliminate many behavioural problems. You must realise that the dog is a pack animal, a member of a social group (*see* Chapter 1), and you, the owners, must be the pack leaders. If this principle is adhered to, as the puppy matures, behavioural problems are unlikely to occur.

Although problems vary from severe aggression to friendly jumping up at people, some are seen more frequently by the veterinary surgeon and these are discussed in this chapter.

AGGRESSION

Apart from that shown by a nervous dog in a situation where his retreat or escape is blocked, aggression is invariably a trait of the dominant dog. The aggression can be directed against *the owner*, *other dogs* or *strangers (territorial aggression)*.

Aggression to Owners

This is shown in dogs who are unsure of their social standing within a family. The aggression may be to all members of the family but it is more usually directed against just one. In our experience, it is usually seen in male dogs with aggression directed at the wife, or children. This behaviour is more commonly seen in the larger breeds which have been specially selected for aggression, such as the Dobermann or Rottweiler, but it can be seen in any breed. This type of dog will often tolerate people outside the immediate family with aggression usually being shown when the dog is challenged or asked to do something. This may be as simple as attempting to move the dog off the sofa or making him leave his basket or a room.

Correction   Reduce the dog's status within the family by everyone cooling their relationship with him. The wolf pack leader does not patrol his pack caressing, fawning and giving attention to his subordinates, so neither should the owner of an aggressive dog. Simply ignore the dog and do not make any approaches to him at all. This applies to all members of the family.

If he approaches and seeks attention, this should be given, thus converting him to the subordinate role. If such attention is sought, the dog should be made to perform a subordinate action such as to sit or to give a paw before being rewarded.

All privileges should be stopped. The dog should not be allowed on to any beds except his own, or any chairs. Perhaps he should even be banned from the family room during the evenings. He should certainly not be carried.

Initially, any conflicts should be avoided but any order given must be carried through or control will never be gained. Therefore, if a conflict develops, the owner *must* win.

The dog should be handled as much as possible. This is a good policy from puppyhood onwards as the vet may have to handle his feet, ears, mouth, tail, etc., in the surgery. This type of handling will assert the owner's dominance, but if the dog is dangerous it is advisable to muzzle him at first.

Establish dominance with obedience training so the dog obeys the owner's commands. Dog training classes help, but may be regarded as a game which ceases when the class ends unless the training is continued at home.

Pulling on the lead is a dominant characteristic, and should be prevented. Dogs pull because they can see what they wish to pull towards. Conventional collars or choke chains do little to help but a Halti will correct this instantly. This is like a miniature horse's halter with a nose band as well as a neck band. The lead attaches to the nose band which closes gently when the lead is pulled. In addition, because the pull is on the muzzle, the dog's head is easily turned towards the direction of pull. It is rather like having power steering on a car! The dog stops pulling because he cannot see what he

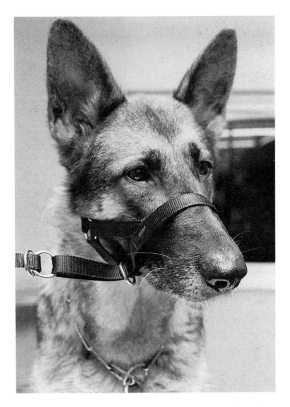

A German Shepherd Dog wearing a Halti.

was pulling towards and feels vulnerable. A Halti is very effective in reducing the dominance of the dog and can be used either as a training device for a few weeks only, or permanently, instead of the usual collar.

Most dominant dogs are male so hormone treatment or castration has a beneficial effect on reducing dominance. This can, and should, be used if other methods fail. Castration has no adverse affects on a male dog; his general non-sexual temperament should not change and, as the operation is performed under a general anaesthetic, the dog is not aware of the procedure. Post-operative recovery is usually straightforward and the patient is back to his five mile walks within about ten days. Occasionally, over-indulgence in food can cause weight gain but this is easily controlled by diet.

Aggression to Other Dogs

To re-train a dog who is aggressive to others, it is necessary to have control of the aggressive dog during attacks and also to punish the attack behaviour and reward desirable behaviour. A very effective method is demonstrated by Dr Roger Mugford, an animal behaviourist. Dr Mugford uses his Red Setter, Sam, as a stooge dog against whom attacks by the patient are thwarted using a few devices. These are:

1 The Halti.
2 A Dog Stop alarm. This alarm is similar to a rape alarm and when pressed, it emits a high-pitched shrill that is particularly un-pleasant for dogs.
3 A retractable flexi-lead with which the dog can be controlled at a distance.

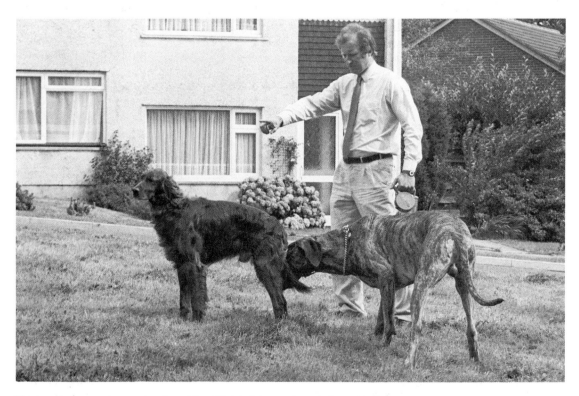

Treatment of aggression to other dogs using a Halti, dog stop alarm and a stooge dog.

The stooge dog should be a very placid, friendly dog whose only wish in life is to play. The attack of the aggressor is interrupted by the shrill alarm and the dog directed gently sideways by the Halti and flexi-lead. At this stage, pleasurable behaviour such as play should be attempted with the aggressor.

This combination of events should be carried out many times until the aggressor is indeed playing with his previously intended victim – often within minutes! In addition, this course of action should be carried out with as many stooge dogs on as many occasions as possible.

It may also be necessary to use hormone treatment or consider castration in the aggressive male dog.

Aggression to Strangers (Territorial Aggression)

This type of aggression is seen in those dogs who have a particularly strong attachment to their owner and territory. It seems to occur mostly in the German Shepherd Dog who has a highly developed sense of owner loyalty. It is not difficult to see how aggression develops in a dog of this type. He is reared and kept in isolation from other dogs and humans, and often not exercised away from his own territory. It can be exaggerated by an early unpleasant encounter with a stranger – dustman, postman, etc. – and even by over-aggressive handling by trainers at classes.

Owning a dog of this type can severely affect the family life-style. Friends may cease visiting, as may the postman, milkman and dustman. In addition, if neighbours and children are bitten, legal action may ensue. It is essential to re-train such a dog if at all possible.

Correction If the dog is dangerous it must be muzzled both to safeguard the public and to aid corrective training.

The dog must be taught that other people are acceptable. Using a Halti and a one metre lead should enable other people to control and walk the dog.

Visitors to the dog's territory must not present a challenge. They should move slowly and as little as possible, speak quietly, not challenge the dog, carry a few dog biscuits, and carry a briefcase, or similar, to act as a shield. On many occasions, we have found ourselves in exactly this situation. This is when the black veterinary bag has come in useful, as have the biscuits in the pocket!

The owner must exert dominance more frequently, particularly when visitors are present. The most submissive gesture on the part of the dog is the down position, lying on his back or side with legs in the air and this should be achieved as often as possible.

Unless re-trained, this type of dog should be kept muzzled whenever contact with strangers is possible, or alternatively kept in secure escape-proof premises.

FIGHTING WITHIN THE PACK

We see this problem particularly in pairs of dogs of the same sex and breed, especially litter mates or mother and female offspring. Indeed, fighting bitches are often worse, as they do not submit as easily as males. As such dogs are almost equally matched, it is not easy for them to sort out the pecking order. The resultant fighting can be very persistent and worrying for the owner and, of course, dangerous for the dogs.

It is essential for one dog to be dominant and one submissive. They will then live in complete harmony. Owners must do all they can to reinforce dominance in the top dog and submissiveness in the subordinate, bearing in mind that, as the family is the pack, so the owners must be dominant to the dogs.

Correction

1 Avoid keeping litter mates of like sexes.

2 Avoid keeping mother/daughter pairs.

3 If the problem occurs, decide which of the dogs is to be the dominant one and then be ruthless and consistent in denying privileges to the underdog. Feed the dominant one first, greet him first, reward him first, let him sit with you, etc.

4 In any tussle, reprimand the underdog, not the dominant one who may appear to have started the argument. By a look or posture, however, it is almost certainly the underdog who challenged him.

5 To start with, you should almost ignore the underdog until the pecking order is established.

6 Hormone treatment may be prescribed by your vet to reduce the dominance of the underdog and, indeed, castration may be recommended in an entire male.

7 The owner should spend plenty of time out with both dogs but at all times he should pay more attention to the intended leader. This teaches the dogs to socialise together.

Correction may be impossible and if a powerful or stubborn breed is involved, such as Bull Terriers or Jack Russells, it may well be necessary to re-home one of the pair. This can be a heart-breaking decision but may be the best way from the *dog's* point of view. Each dog individually will be a delightful pet, either as an only pet or with another dog dissimilar to himself. It is, therefore, foolish (and possibly dangerous) to put up with a permanent, explosive situation rather than make this sensible decision. The difficulty is in deciding which one of a pair has to go and here your vet may be able to advise you.

NERVOUS DOGS

Most dogs are well balanced, slightly extrovert individuals who find it easy to socialise and respond to other dogs and people. A few, however, are excessively shy and retiring and find the world a worrying place. Hiding away reduces the stress of socialising, the dog feels safer and so hides more often. A nervous dog hiding in a corner or other safe place can become defensively aggressive if attempts are made to extract him from his safe area.

Correction The earlier in the dog's life correction is started the better, so that the benefits of hiding away are not fully learnt.

The dog may pull excessively on a choke chain, causing distress and pain. A collar may slip off in the struggle, so a Halti may well be a gentler way of preventing retreat and moving the dog towards you. Reward the dog's approach to you with titbits and praise, and punish retreat by voice or with a water pistol.

Once the decision to re-train the dog has been taken, a consistent, extrovert approach on the part of the owner will help. In other words, do not sympathise with the dog. A common scenario in our hospital is a nervous dog, cowering in the corner of the consulting room, with the owner kneeling beside him saying 'Be a good boy' and trying to tempt him out. This is a mistake because the dog interprets 'good boy' as a reward which reinforces the nervous behaviour and makes matters worse.

Instead, try a totally new outgoing approach to life and this will often stun the dog into joining in. This type of approach is often easier with total strangers where a strict approach often works because the dog realises the familiar, soothing responses of the owner are not forthcoming.

Drug therapy will help in some cases and drugs may be prescribed by your vet.

DESTRUCTIVE DOGS

Apart from the chewing carried out by puppies in an attempt to soothe painful teeth, most destructiveness by dogs is due to anxiety at being separated from their owners. This separation may be merely by one room but more usually it is when the dog is left in the house or car on its own. Occasionally, the motive may be fury at being disciplined or just sheer loneliness, as the dog is a very social species.

Correction

1 Prevent access to the environment by using an indoor or outdoor kennel.
2 Muzzle the dog for short periods in the car or house.
3 Avoid boredom by leaving the dog with toys to play with, especially those suitable for chewing such as large raw marrow bones or tough chewing toys such as 'Kongs'. It may help to provide the dog with a box full of toys just as you are about to leave the house.
4 Exercise the dog just before leaving. He may then feel happy to lie down and sleep for a while.
5 Similarly, feed the dog before leaving. Sleep may be induced on a full stomach.
6 Leave the house in an occupied condition — warm, with the lights and radio on.
7 Avoid exaggerated departures as this increases the dog's anxiety when you leave by raising his joy at your attention prior to leaving. It is far better to slip out almost unnoticed, avoiding any fuss.
8 A general cooling of the relationship between dog and owner will help to reduce the separation anxiety when leaving the house. In other words, if being with the owner is suddenly not so much fun, then being without the owner is not so bad.
9 Devote some time to disorientation of the dog, retraining and confusing him over how long you will be away. Leave and return in about a minute, stay a while and then leave and return in about ten minutes. Vary this routine over a whole day or several days until the dog can tolerate longer periods of separation.

Drug therapy may be helpful, if all else fails. The diazepam compounds (Valium) can be useful in certain cases and may be prescribed by your vet.

The problem can usually be avoided if puppies are trained at an early age to be separated from their owners for gradually increasing lengths of time.

BAD TRAVELLERS

This includes both the excitable whining traveller and the nervous dog who feels nauseated by car travel.

Excitable Whining Dogs

This usually starts when the dog realises that a car ride is the prelude to a walk and becomes excited too early. It can be extremely distressing and dangerous to the owner/driver.

Correction Keep the dog's head below window level so that exciting stimuli are not appreciated. This can be done by sitting the dog on the floor of the car and possibly keeping him there on a short lead. Distract his attention with something like a water pistol or Dog Stop shrill alarm when he starts whining.

A travelling kennel in the car may help to avoid the visual stimuli. In extreme cases, it may be necessary to consider exchanging the car for a van.

Nervous, Travel-Sick Dogs

Such dogs, in contrast to the previous type, are usually reluctant to even enter the car.

Thus, a useful first step is to convince the dog that the car is a pleasant place in which to be. Feed the dog in the stationary car and play with him there, or just sit and read while the dog sleeps. Entice the dog to run through the car in the drive with the doors open by throwing toys, such as rubber rings, through the car. When the dog is happy with the above, try them all with the engine running, but the car still stationary.

To start with, drive the car only a hundred metres or so. Then gradually extend the length of the journeys as the dog becomes used to the car. Ensure the journey always ends with a treat, such as a walk or a meal.

As a last resort, short-term drug treatment to either depress anxiety or control vomiting may be prescribed by your vet.

THE OVERSEXED MALE DOG

Many puppies on reaching puberty will experiment with 'mating' chairs, bean bags, legs, children and other dogs. This is a normal phase and in most cases will pass.

Some dogs, however, continue with this anti-social habit despite the most rigorous correction. It is, of course, misplaced normal behaviour and under more natural circumstances, with mates available, the dog would not indulge in this aberrant activity. Apart from the anti-social nature of the habit, it can be dangerous as young children can be overbalanced and pushed to the ground.

Treatment Medical treatment using hormones will often help a young adult dog through this phase. Corrective training while receiving hormones may be all that is needed.

If, however, despite treatment the dog continues to be oversexed, surgical castration is the treatment preferred. This operation should be carried out as soon as possible for maximum effect once it has been recommended. In our opinion, it is kinder to the dog to castrate him and remove the strong desire to mate, rather than to leave him entire, frustrated and not allowed to mate for the whole of his life. The operation to remove his testicles is performed through a very small incision under a general anaesthetic. Recovery is normally rapid and smooth, the dog showing no after-effects or awareness of the nature of the operation.

TOILET TRAINING

Two types of toilet training problem exist. These are the territorial urination of the adult, sexually excited, male dog and the failure to learn the correct site for urination and defaecation.

Territorial Urination

The wild fox will urinate and defaecate at positions within and around his territory, both to attract mates and warn off competitors. An oversexed male dog will sometimes feel the need to do likewise and his territory may include the lounge, sofa and carpets. Although this is usually a problem of the male dog, we have known female transgressors also.

Correction No amount of training will correct this. It is necessary to resort to drug therapy with hormone treatment. Frequently, castration of the male dog is necessary before the problem is resolved.

The problem occurs more often where there is a challenge to the male dog in the form of a new dog in the household or even a new neighbour's dog. Removal of the unwanted interloper will often resolve the problem.

House Training

Normal Puppy Training

The puppy will be taught by his dam to leave the nest to urinate and defaecate. At eight weeks old he will be able to control his bladder and bowels for a few seconds to enable him to do this. Gradually, this period lengthens and by ten to twelve weeks, you should be able to recognise the actions and expressions which mean the puppy is about to toilet – circling with a worried expression. Now is the time to pick him up and take him to the desired place, the garden if it is dry and somewhere like the porch if it is wet. On wet days, use newspaper as a last resort but remember that before long, newspaper will not be acceptable to you.

Reward every toilet episode in the correct place enthusiastically and slightly reprimand every misdemeanour – but *only* if you catch the puppy in the act.

A puppy usually urinates and defaecates immediately after feeding, so be ready to take him straight outside after a meal. Also, on waking after a sleep puppies usually need to relieve themselves, so this usually means a very early rise at about 6 a.m. for several weeks for the owner of a new puppy.

This effort to house train is well worthwhile for once the puppy is in a routine of waking and going straight outside, as bladder and bowel control improves he will recognise that he has to wait until he is able

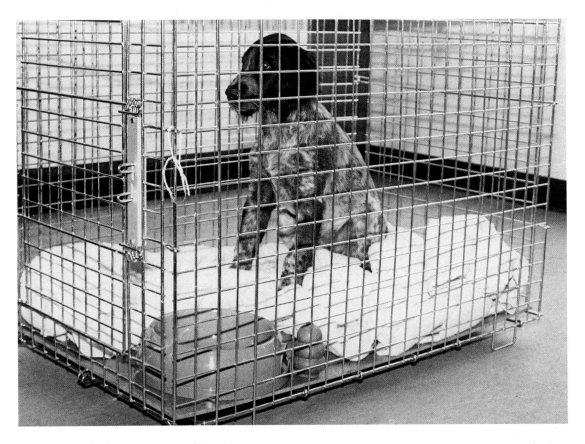

A large Munsterlander puppy in a portable training crate.

to go outside. Gradually, the puppy will associate the reward with toileting in the correct place and the message will get through.

If a catch phrase such as 'off you go' is used when training the puppy to perform, this will develop into a command with the puppy performing to order. This is extremely useful because as well as ensuring the puppy toilets in the right place, it also means he toilets at the right time. This can be very useful when holidaying in hotels or on campsites.

Very few puppies are completely house-trained before three months of age but most are by eight months.

Correction of Toileting Problems of the Older Puppy or Dog

Feed a diet which leaves a low residue and is mostly absorbed by the dog. Less fibre means less bulky motions.

The smell of urine and faeces stimulates the dog to perform, so proper cleaning of soiled areas is necessary. Ammonia-based disinfectants must be avoided as these smell like urine to the dog. Either biological detergents or proprietary enzyme products available from your vet or pet shop should be used to eliminate these smells.

A dog will usually defaecate within eight hours of eating. Thus, dogs which defaecate overnight should be fed in the morning and those which defaecate in the house in the daytime, while the owner is away, should be fed at night. This will minimise the chance of mistakes. The dog should be allowed frequent access to the garden or toileting area, and rewarded when he performs.

As dogs will rarely soil the bed, an indoor cage or kennel can be used successfully to confine him while the owner is not directly observing him. On release, he will often perform immediately on command in the proper place and should be justly rewarded.

The use of a catch-phrase every time he performs will usually lead to a word association response. Dogs trained in this way will defaecate or urinate on command. This, of course, is a great advantage and perfectly simple to achieve.

COPROPHAGY (FAECES EATING)

To humans, this is a most abhorrent habit of dogs but in fact it causes them no harm at all. However, it is the behavioural problem on which our advice is most often sought.

In the young, rapidly growing puppy, faeces can provide a source of both vitamins and fat, and a puppy's natural curiosity often leads him to experiment. As it is an undesirable habit, steps must be taken to correct it, and an attentive owner will of course do so. It usually only becomes a problem when it develops into a habit as a result of lack of supervision or correction. Active breeds, such as Labradors, show this behaviour most commonly, especially those in a kennel situation.

Correction

1 Train the puppy to defaecate on demand, and pick up and dispose of faeces immediately to make sure the puppy cannot reach them again.
2 Ensure the correct diet is fed, containing enough nutrients and energy. Vitamin and mineral supplements are useful.
3 Increase the fibre content of the diet to make the puppy feel more full. This can be done by adding bran or grated raw carrot.
4 Ensure the puppy is thoroughly wormed to prevent the depraved appetite that parasitic worms can cause.
5 Deliver a severe verbal reprimand each time the puppy is caught eating faeces.

If all else fails, there are some food additives which may render the faeces unpalatable. Sodium monoglutamate, iron compounds and amino acids are among those tried with varying degrees of success but your vet should be consulted first.

THE OLDER DOG

Finally, a word of warning about obtaining an older dog as a new pet. A puppy of six to twelve weeks old will grow up used to your way of life. An older dog in need of a new home may well suit your every need but, of course, he may have been trained to a totally different type of household and family. As a simple illustration, the original owner may have had a job which entailed getting up at 5 a.m. which is when the dog was let out to toilet. The dog may continue to expect this for the rest of his life. It is essential to discuss fully the dog's temperament and behaviour with the previous owner or stray-home superintendent before purchasing such an older dog. If these simple precautions are taken, an older dog with none of the tricky house training problems may turn out to be the ideal pet.

18 First Aid, Accidents and Emergencies

First Aid is the emergency treatment of a dog suffering from the effects of an accident or sudden illness before full veterinary medical and surgical help is available. The primary objectives of First Aid are to keep the dog alive, to preserve his health and strength and to make him comfortable, until he can be seen by a vet.

PRIORITIES IN AN EMERGENCY

1 **Stay calm.** If you panic you merely impair your own performance and become illogical.

2 **Contact the vet as soon as possible.** He will be able to advise you on your immediate action. He may ask you to bring the dog to the surgery immediately, in which case he will make the necessary preparations. The vet may, on the other hand, decide to visit the injured dog.

3 **Protect yourself from injury.** A shocked and painful dog may bite anyone so use a muzzle or a blanket to avoid this.

4 **Control haemorrhage.** Severe haemorrhage must be controlled, regardless of other injuries.

5 **Clear the dog's airways.** Pull the tongue forward, away from the back of the throat, clearing away any fluid such as vomit or blood.

6 **Let him lie as he wants to.**

TRANSPORT OF THE INJURED DOG

Few emergencies can be treated as effectively in the home or on the roadside as at the surgery. Thus, it makes total sense to transport an acutely ill dog to the veterinary surgery in the same way as an ambulance takes an injured person to hospital. However, care must be taken in moving injured dogs in order to avoid worsening the situation.

A small dog can be gently lifted in the owner's arms and driven to the surgery. It is advisable to lift him in a blanket, both for support in case of leg or spinal injury and to protect the owner from bite wounds. A larger dog, or one where fractures are suspected, may be gently manoeuvred onto a blanket or board and lifted into the car by a person holding each end. It may be necessary to muzzle him first.

Having alerted the veterinary surgeon, you should then drive steadily and carefully to ensure the dog is not subjected to sudden movements.

SHOCK

Shock is a complicated and serious clinical syndrome which leads to an inadequate blood supply to vital organs. If uncorrected, death can and does occur. It is shock, not fractures, that is the major cause of death after road accidents, and the likelihood of delayed shock is the reason that most vets will suggest a thorough examination and

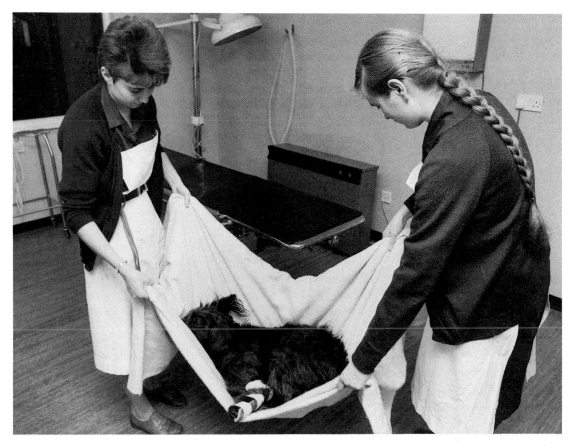

Transport of an injured dog using a blanket.

usually a short stay in the surgery for a road accident victim.

Signs of Shock

1 Unconsciousness or extreme weakness.
2 Pale gums.
3 Skin feels cold as do extremities such as ears.
4 A rapid heartbeat and weak pulse.
5 Rapid shallow breathing.

Causes of Shock

Shock is usually caused by a massive decrease in blood volume usually as a result of haemorrhage which may, of course, not be apparent if the bleeding is internal. It can also be caused by the large fluid loss caused by burns and scalds. Severe stress or trauma such as the extensive injuries and pain following a road accident can also lead to shock.

First Aid Treatment of Shock

Firstly, ensure that breathing continues. Clear the airway and, if necessary, give mouth-to-mouth resuscitation by cupping the muzzle in your hands and blowing down the nostril twenty times a minute.

If the heart appears to have stopped, external massage by pressing the chest between your hands, with the dog lying on his side, should be attempted. This should be at the rate of sixty times per minute.

Haemorrhage must be controlled as any further blood loss may be critical. Blood loss

217

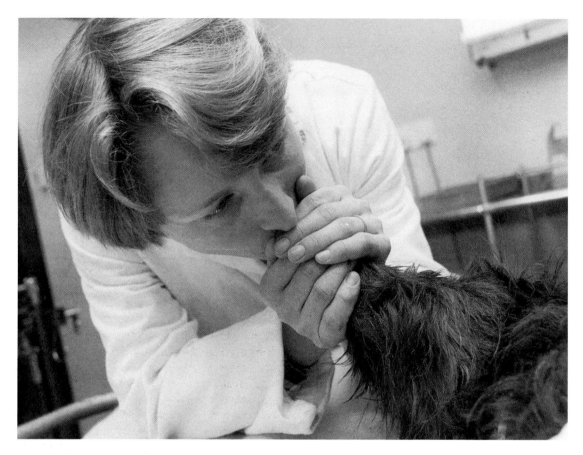

Mouth to mouth resuscitation of an unconscious dog.

from arteries is bright red and spurts rhythmically whereas blood from veins flows freely and is darker. Capillary blood loss oozes into the wound. A tourniquet can be made out of a clean cloth or a tie, and should be applied above the wound. Direct pressure on the haemorrhaging wound, using a clean cloth, is very helpful and a bandage can be applied over this to help stop the bleeding.

The dog must also be wrapped in a blanket or a coat to keep him warm. Lie the dog on his side, with his head lower than the rest of his body to encourage the flow of blood to the brain.

The Veterinary Surgeon's Approach to Shock

As the main cause of shock is lowering of the circulating blood volume, the vet will correct this as a matter of priority. A plasma substitute or whole blood, if available, will be administered as a transfusion, dripped slowly into a vein usually in the dog's foreleg. It will normally be necessary for the dog to be hospitalised for this procedure as a transfusion may take hours, during which time he must be monitored closely by a vet or veterinary nurse.

Warmth from an infra-red lamp or electric blanket should be provided, together with adequate bedding to prevent heat loss.

If breathing is severely impaired in the

throat, the vet may have to perform a tracheotomy, whereby an opening is created directly into the trachea.

SPECIFIC ACCIDENTS AND EMERGENCIES

The Road Accident

This is perhaps the most wide-ranging emergency because it can involve several different life threatening injuries at the same time.

Unconsciousness

Lay the dog on his side and pull out the tongue to ensure the airway is clear. Check

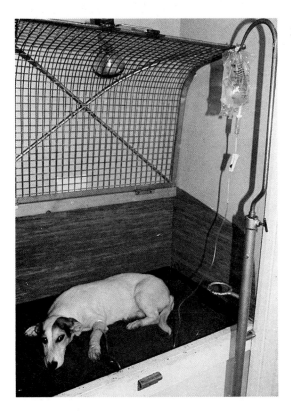

A dog in shock receiving an intravenous fluid transfusion.

the dog is breathing. A wet finger in front of the nostril is a good test if you are uncertain.

Haemorrhage and Shock

Shock should be minimised by controlling haemorrhage (described more fully under shock, *see* page 216), and preventing heat loss by using a blanket or coat.

Bone Fractures

A fracture is a broken bone. It is highly likely that one or more fractures will result from an impact with a car, so care must be taken in lifting and transporting such a patient. Fractures usually occur in the legs and pelvis, but they are also seen in the spine, skull and ribs. A fracture of one of the lower bones of a leg may be obvious. The leg will often protrude at a strange angle below the break. If possible, this should be gently straightened and secured with bandage, tape or string to a splint made out of a piece of wood, or rolled-up newspaper, magazines or cardboard. If it is impossible to correct the angle, then support the leg so it cannot move further.

A fracture of the upper bones of the front or hind leg, or pelvis is more difficult to both diagnose and support. If such a fracture is suspected, the dog should be allowed to lie as he pleases and be transported gently.

If a spinal fracture is suspected by, perhaps, paralysis of the hind legs or obvious deformity of the spine, the dog must be moved with great care and transported on a board or door.

Dislocations

First Aid for dislocations is identical to that of suspected fracture. Prompt treatment is essential for the vet to restore the leg to full function.

219

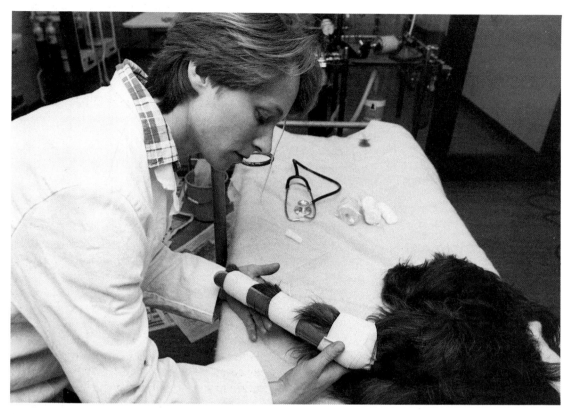

A temporary splint being applied to the foreleg of a road accident victim.

Dog Fights

The priority here is to separate the dogs without injury to either people or dogs. A distraction is essential - merely reaching for your own dog's collar will often result in a bite from an already suspicious and excited dog. Shouting may help, as may soaking the dogs in water or the use of a loud whistle. Hitting one, or both, dogs with a rolled up newspaper may help. Another effective method we have used is to lift both hind feet of one dog and pull him away while the other one is controlled by his owner.

Quite horrific injuries can result due to the length of the dog's canine (tearing) teeth. These can fracture bones, penetrate joints or cause huge gaping wounds.

Action Control any haemorrhage and bathe wounds with warm sterile water or dilute antiseptic to remove debris. Bandage open wounds to prevent further haemorrhage and infection.

As dogs' teeth invariably carry bacteria through the skin in any penetrating wound, infection often follows a bite wound. Abscesses may result, especially in small but deep puncture wounds. An antibiotic injection administered by the vet at the time of the bite should prevent this. Larger wounds may require sutures and should be protected until examined by the vet.

Prolapsed Eyeball

This will often follow a fight and is usually seen in short-nosed breeds such as Pekes and Pugs. The eye is forced out of its socket, and the lids clamp shut behind it. Unless it is replaced within fifteen minutes, the sight and even the eye are invariably lost due to swelling caused by constriction of the blood vessels supplying the eye.

Action As speed is essential, the person in charge of the dog should attempt to replace the eyeball. One person should pull the eyelids apart while another, using moist sterile gauze or soft cloth, gently presses on the eye ball to replace it back in the socket. If this is impossible, the eyeball should be kept covered with this moist sterile gauze and the dog taken to the vet immediately.

Burns and Scalds

The immediate action should be to cool the skin down using cold running water if possible. Do not apply any ointments or lotions. After this initial action, cold compresses should be applied to affected areas and the dog should be kept quiet and prevented from making the injury worse by biting and scratching.

Burns can result from causes other than direct heat or hot water. Friction burns commonly occur after road accidents. Chemical burns can occur after contact with corrosive chemicals such as paraffin, turpentine, acids, etc., and should be thoroughly irrigated with sterile water to wash away any remains of the chemical.

The dog should be taken to the vet as soon as possible to ensure shock does not occur and to prevent damage and infection of the burn wound.

Electrocution

This is usually a problem of the inquisitive, bored puppy who chews through a live electric cable.

Action If the puppy is unconscious and lying near a chewed cable, switch off the electricity first or you may also be electrocuted. It may be sensible to push him away

from the wire or appliances with a brush, for instance.

Only then, if the dog is unconscious, begin artificial respiration and external heart massage as described under shock (*see* page 216).

Foreign Bodies

Ball in Throat

This occurs when the dog is playing with a ball that is too small. It becomes lodged behind the tongue in the pharynx and is too large to be swallowed and too far back for the tongue to remove. It acts literally as a ball-valve and is an acute emergency which we see several times a year. The dog becomes frantic, salivates profusely, paws at his mouth and is obviously in respiratory distress. As we write this, one of our patients, a magnificent German Shepherd Dog, has just died from this condition within seconds, in front of his distressed owner while playing in the park with a squash ball. There was no time for her even to telephone our hospital for help.

Action Do not attempt to remove the ball by reaching inside the mouth as you will only push it further in. Instead, try to press on the underside of the back of the throat from the outside and push the ball upwards and forwards. It should move over the back of the tongue, and the dog will cough it out.

If this is not possible, then drive straight to the nearest vet and try to give the dog plenty of air. He must be kept very still to minimise his use of oxygen, and the emergency must be dealt with the instant you arrive at the surgery. Despite the life-threatening nature of this condition, we have been successful in resolving many emergencies of this type over the years.

Foreign Body in Mouth

This is a frequent emergency and is usually due to a stick or bone becoming wedged between the teeth. Often it will be wedged across the roof of the mouth between the left and right upper teeth when the dog bites on it, although bones, especially small cooked chop bones, may wedge between adjacent teeth at the back of the mouth.

The dog suddenly starts to salivate and paw at his mouth, and he will often chew frantically. His breathing may be noisy due to excess saliva and obstruction of the air flow.

Action The foreign body should be removed either with your fingers or with a pair of pliers. It may be helpful to put a wooden object between his canine teeth so you can search the mouth safely and remove the offending object.

Fish-Hooks

If a dog chews a fish with a hook in it, the hook may become caught in the dog's mouth or swallowed into the stomach. Occasionally, the fish-hook may become caught in the skin.

Action If you can reach the fish-hook, wherever it is, do not try to pull it out. Either push it through the skin, or cut the hook anywhere on its length with pliers, pincers or a hacksaw and then push the barbed end through.

If you cannot remove the hook, take the dog to the vet. If the fishing line leads into the mouth and disappears behind the tongue, do not pull it. Leave it in place and take him to the vet. *Do not cut the line* or the vet may not be able to trace the hook.

Grass Seeds

In the summer and autumn, seeds of the wild barley lodge in the hair, especially in the coat of long-haired breeds such as the Cocker Spaniel. The symptoms shown depend on the site of the seed.

In the ear or on the ear flap, the seed will cause sudden violent shaking of the head during, or shortly after, a walk. Elsewhere on the body a sore area may develop, leading to a small abscess. This is particularly common between the toes and will also lead to lameness. In the eye, the seed often lodges behind the third eyelid and causes pain and discharge. Usually only one eye is affected.

Action If a grass seed is suspected, search very carefully and if one is located, remove it. You may need a pair of tweezers. If you cannot remove it do not ignore it but take the dog to a vet. These seeds act like a fish-hook because of their shape, and can only move one way – inwards. They will penetrate intact skin and, if neglected, can migrate long distances within the body. We have seen one that entered between the toes and after causing severe abscessation for over a year, eventually came out at the elbow when the problem immediately cleared up.

Foreign Body in Pad

Glass fragments, thorns, or splinters will often penetrate the pad of the foot and cause pain and lameness. A careful search of the pad may reveal the object or, more likely, a tell-tale small wet opening which is acutely painful when pressed. The foreign body will have penetrated the hardened skin of the pad and will be lodged in the soft sensitive tissues below.

Action To remove the foreign body, use a sharp needle sterilised in a flame or spirit and gently enlarge the opening in the dead skin of the pad by picking at the hole. The dog cannot feel this. Do not insert the needle into the pad at all. When the hole has been enlarged, place one thumb either side of the hole, press gently and move the thumbs away from each other, thereby opening the hole a little. The foreign body will often pop out. If not, take the dog along to the vet as an anaesthetic may be needed.

Lead Clip on Foot

This occurs with the spring-type lead clip when the dog accidentally steps heavily on his lead. It is very difficult to remove, as pressing on the spring merely tightens the clip against the web of the foot, causing pain.

Action To remove the clip, use a hacksaw or wire clippers and cut through the spring. Then, buy a lead with a better type of clip! Sometimes, the web is so swollen and painful that a general anaesthetic is needed.

Snake Bite

Do not attempt First Aid. Take the dog to a vet as quickly as possible.

Bee and Wasp Stings

These are usually a problem of young playful puppies in the summer. The sting frequently occurs in or around the mouth or front feet and is seen as a suddenly appearing, soft, painful swelling. The dog will paw at his mouth or lick his foot.

Action Wasps withdraw their sting after an attack and move on to pastures new. Their sting is alkaline so bathe with a dilute acid such as vinegar or lemon juice. Bees sting once only and leave the sting in the dog. Look for the sting and remove it from

the dog with tweezers. It looks like a thick, dark, short hair with a tiny bit of flesh on the free end. Bee stings are acidic so bathe with a mild alkaline such as bicarbonate of soda.

If the dog is very distressed, a vet will give him an antihistamine injection to counteract the sting.

Heatstroke

This is an acute emergency which we frequently see in hot weather. It usually occurs in dogs that have been shut in cars with insufficient ventilation. In a closed car on a summer day when the temperature is, say, 21°C (70°F) the greenhouse effect

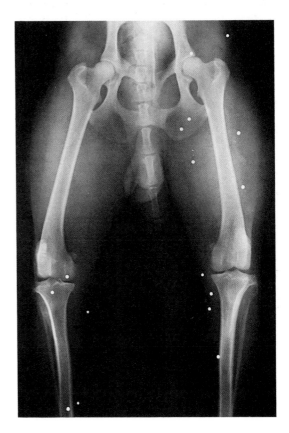

This Springer Spaniel was shot accidentally. The X-ray shows numerous pieces of lead shot present in the leg and rump.

rapidly increases the temperature inside the car to over 38°C (101°F). Within minutes, the dog is in severe distress and can die very rapidly. Even with windows open, dogs should not be shut in cars on hot days. On cooler days the windows must be left open and grills fitted.

Action A heatstroke victim will be severely distressed, frantically panting and may be collapsed. His temperature will be greatly elevated, 41°C (106°F) or more, so he must be placed immediately into a cold bath or river, or be hosed down with water instead. His temperature should be taken every three minutes and when it reaches the normal 38.6°C (101.5°F) he should be dried and put in a cool place. At all stages water, preferably with salt added at the rate of one teaspoonful per half litre, should be available for him to drink.

If he does not recover rapidly, take him to the vet as he may be suffering from shock.

Convulsions or Fits

The commonest cause of convulsions is **epilepsy**. The dog suddenly loses control, starts to champ at the jaws and salivates. He then collapses and lies on his side with all four legs either rigid or twitching. He may, or may not, howl at the same time. This fit is usually over within two to five minutes, after which the dog is subdued for a while but rapidly returns to normal. Fits can occur either singly or as a series, one after the other. (*See also* Chapter 13, page 167).

Action The immediate First Aid is to prevent him from damaging himself during the fit so he should be gently but firmly held down. When the fit is over, you should telephone the vet's surgery for an appointment, or take him along to the next open surgery. There is no need to panic as fits do not usually last very long. However, if the fits

occur in rapid succession, or the dog does not recover from a fit within a few minutes, there may be a more serious reason and the vet should be contacted without delay. A common cause of suddenly occurring, continuous fits is poisoning by slug pellets, which contain metaldehyde, and veterinary treatment is essential.

There are other causes of fits apart from epilepsy so your vet may need to investigate the problem further, taking blood tests or X-rays.

Eclampsia

Eclampsia, or milk fever, is an emergency that occurs in a bitch who is suckling puppies. It usually, but not always, occurs at the period of maximum demand on her milk supply when the puppies are about three weeks old. It is caused by a dramatic lowering of the calcium level in her bloodstream which has been used up in the huge milk supply to the puppies.

The bitch starts to behave a little oddly, then to twitch and stagger a little. Within about half an hour she begins to convulse and it is essential she is taken to a vet without delay, or the condition will prove fatal.

Action There is no First Aid once the bitch is showing symptoms and the vet must be contacted without delay. Treatment usually consists of the injection of a calcium solution, either into the vein (intravenously) or under the skin (subcutaneously) depending on her condition. The puppies should be weaned immediately.

Prevention should be attempted by ensuring an adequate calcium supply during pregnancy and lactation.

Heart Attacks

Fortunately heart attacks rarely occur in dogs, as heart disease in the dog does not involve a sudden blockage of the coronary arteries and a resulting heart attack. Heart murmurs are the common cause of heart disease and these will lead to cardiac insufficiency. If an affected dog overdoes it, he may black out or faint and this acts as a safety valve. Once the dog is rested, he will usually regain consciousness within minutes.

Action Wrap the dog in a blanket and lay him on his side. Gentle massage of the chest helps to stimulate the circulation. In small breeds, pressure over the heart is achieved using the finger and thumb on either side of the rib cage, while in larger breeds, it is easier to compress the chest rhythmically either between the hands, or between the hands and a table or floor.

A drop of brandy on the back of the tongue will often cause the dog to gasp and take in oxygen which should revive him. He should then be examined by a vet.

Epistaxis (Nose Bleed)

This is seen as a sudden haemorrhage from the nose. It is usually caused by trauma or violent sneezing.

Action First Aid is aimed at making the blood clot where it is haemorrhaging. The dog should be kept quiet. Ice packs or cold cloths placed over the nose can speed up clotting. It also helps to lift the nose so that it points upwards. If the bleeding does not cease rapidly, the vet should be contacted.

Paraphimosis

This is a prolonged erection of the penis which is unable to retract back into the sheath after mating or attempted mating. It very swollen due to the constriction of the base caused by the sheath and can be very difficult to replace.

The exposed penis should be protected by gently bathing it in cool sterile water. This may reduce it in size and enable you to move the sheath forward over it. Lubrication may be necessary using petroleum jelly or soap, after which it should be possible to pull the sheath gently forwards to enclose the penis. If correction proves impossible veterinary help is needed.

Gastric Dilatation and Torsion

This is the canine equivalent of bloat in cattle and sheep and it is an extremely serious emergency. The stomach distends rapidly with gas, usually a very frothy gas that the dog cannot eliminate. It will then often twist, thereby effectively closing the entrance and exit to the stomach. This is called a gastric torsion. There is now no escape for the gases and the stomach rapidly distends to fill the entire abdomen. The skin in the area is under great tension and resembles a drum skin.

The dog rapidly becomes pear-shaped and has great difficulty in breathing due to pressure on the diaphragm. His gums and tongue turn greyish blue due to circulatory failure, and shock rapidly follows. The dog is obviously in distress and should be taken to the veterinary surgeon immediately.

Action The dog is unlikely to survive unless he has veterinary attention within half an hour of the onset of severe symptoms.

Avoid gastric dilatation and torsion by taking care not to exercise your dog for about an hour after a full meal. This is especially important in deep-chested breeds such as German Shepherd Dogs, Great Danes, Setters and Boxers.

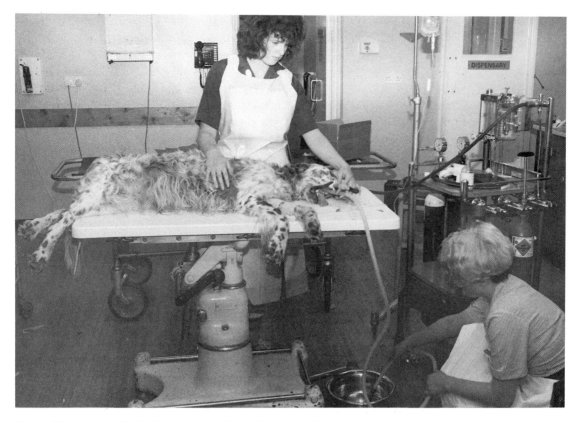

Gastric dilatation in an English Setter. A stomach tube is being used to empty the stomach of the fermenting contents.

Poisonings

Dogs can be poisoned by a multitude of substances, either accidentally or deliberately. The source can be poisonous plants (indoor or outdoor), chemicals such as pesticides, antifreeze, paint, or drugs that the owner may be taking.

Action   If the dog has been seen to take the suspected poison, the most effective treatment is to make the dog sick immediately. Your vet has an injection available, called apomorphine, that will make the dog sick within about a minute and this may be the best approach.

However, it may be worth an attempt to make the dog sick at home. A teaspoonful of table salt placed on the back of the tongue will often induce vomiting, as will a similar amount of washing soda. If an acid has been swallowed give an alkali such as baking soda, or if an alkali has been swallowed give an acid such as vinegar or lemon juice. Copious amounts of water should also be given.

Poisoning is difficult to diagnose because of the many different symptoms, most of which are vague and non-specific. The dog may become excitable or depressed, he may become weak and incoordinated, he may vomit or have diarrhoea. Salivation will often occur; abdominal pain, convulsions and shock may follow.

In any case of suspected poisoning, it is essential to contact the vet as soon as possible. If you know what the dog has eaten, take the packet along or write down the ingredients for the vet. He may then have an antidote to use. The label on the product may have antidotes or First Aid instructions listed.

There are a few specific poisons that are more commonly seen in dogs.

Warfarin

A rat poison. This causes bleeding by preventing blood clotting. An antidote (vitamin K) is available and the dog should be treated by the vet without delay.

Alphachloralose

A rat, mouse and bird poison. The dog becomes weak and collapsed but if kept warm and quiet usually recovers.

Slug Bait (Metaldehyde)

Dogs seem to seek out these small pellets put out to kill slugs. They are very toxic to dogs. Symptoms are weakness and continuous convulsions. There is no specific antidote but the vet will use drugs to counteract the fits and by giving fluids and food intravenously, he may be able to save the dog. (*See* Chapter 13, page 166).

Drugs

Dogs, like children, will investigate containers of tablets left lying around. It is essential to store these correctly. If you suspect your dog of eating these, contact the vet with the name of the drug and he will be able to inform you of the risk and what to do.

Veterinary surgeons have reference books and poison antidotes listed and they also have the knowledge and ability to telephone various Poison Information Centres for advice. Any case of suspected poisoning should be dealt with by a vet to give the dog the maximum chance of survival.

19 The Old Dog

If the dog population is divided into sevenths, we find an interesting distribution of age groups. One seventh are puppies, four sevenths are mature adults, and two sevenths are old dogs. Thus, almost one third of the current population is old and this proportion is certain to increase as veterinary knowledge continues to increase. The care of the older dog is, therefore, an important aspect of both ownership and veterinary practice.

LIFESPAN

It is usually assumed that one year of a dog's life is equivalent to seven of a human. This is a reasonable rule of thumb for the middle-aged dog but a more accurate comparison would be obtained using the table below.

DOG		HUMAN
1	YEAR	15
3	YEAR	30
6	YEAR	40
9	YEAR	55
12	YEAR	65
15	YEAR	80

This, however, is still only a rough guide as the ageing process varies enormously with the breed of dog. In general, smaller breeds live much longer than larger breeds. For instance, an Irish Wolfhound is getting old at eight years, whereas a Jack Russell of fifteen often manages a long walk each day.

GERIATRIC CARE AND DIET

Provided the dog has been well cared for throughout his life and kept fit and in trim, there may be no need to treat him any differently as old age approaches. All dogs should have an annual health check, usually at the time of the vaccination booster, so that any emerging problem can be detected and corrected at an early stage. When the dog reaches ten years old it is sensible to consider more frequent checks by the vet. The extent of these checks will depend on the condition of the dog and the requirements of the owner.

The routine clinical examination of a dog normally takes the vet five to fifteen minutes to complete. During this time he can take his temperature, check his eyes, ears, mouth, skin and coat, chest, abdomen, bones and joints and assess his general condition. If no obvious abnormality is detected, or behavioural change described by the owner, it should not be necessary to take the examination further. If, however, there is reason to suspect the beginnings of organ failure, the vet will probably take blood samples which will reveal whether, for example, the liver and kidneys are functioning normally or beginning to fail. Appropriate action can then be taken to minimise the problem.

It would be sensible to consider six-monthly health checks after the age of ten, increasing to quarterly health checks at the age of fourteen. If your dog suffers from a particular problem, then obviously your vet will advise you on the frequency of visits. We have as patients some healthy old dogs

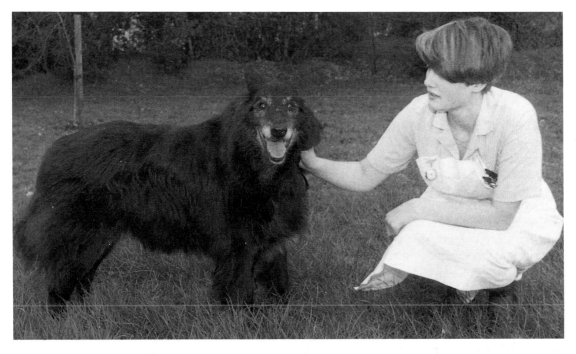

A healthy old Belgian Shepherd Dog.

that come to see us merely once a year, but we also examine others with, say, heart and circulation problems much more frequently. A routine health check every month or two, in some cases, enables us to monitor their progress and amend drug therapy and dosages. This results in healthier patients and less worried owners.

Provided there are no signs of disease or organ deterioration, the most important considerations as old age approaches are diet, fitness and bodily condition.

Diet

The aim should be to feed a diet which will improve existing problems and slow or prevent the development of disease. This diet should enable the dog to maintain his ideal body weight and should also be highly palatable and digestible. It should contain an increased amount of fatty acids, vitamins (especially A, B and E) and certain minerals,

notably zinc. It should, however, contain reduced amounts of protein, phosphorus and sodium and your vet will often recommend a salt-free light diet for older dogs. An appropriate tinned or dried prescription diet is available from your vet or you can make up your own from the following recipe.

Ingredients

115g (4oz) minced meat
1 large hard-boiled egg
75g (3 slices) white bread
350g (12oz) boiled unsalted rice
A balanced vitamin and mineral supplement
(ask your vet for his recommendation)

Method

Braise the meat and use any of the fat produced. Crumble the bread and mix it with all the other ingredients. If it is too

229

dry, moisten with a little water. This produces just over half a kilo of food. It is a complete diet and should be fed in amounts comparable to a normal diet for your dog. Fresh water should, of course, be available at all times but nothing else should be added to the diet.

FITNESS AND EXERCISE

Provided your dog has kept fit with daily walks, there is no need to change the frequency or length of these walks as he becomes older. Apart from the extremely large (giant) breeds, an otherwise healthy dog should hardly need to reduce his exercise routine at all, until he is over ten years old. Many dogs will continue to enjoy long walks until they are over twelve years old. The important point to emphasise is that there should be no change in routine; a sudden drop in exercise is as wrong as a sudden increase in exercise.

The underlying principle is to let the dog tell you when he has had enough exercise. If he lags behind, seems less enthusiastic, has difficulty in walking or getting to his feet after a long walk, or begins to pant excessively on exercise, then it is time to consider less exercise and a health check. Dogs are no different from people in their requirements as they become older – a good diet, company, creature comforts and a change of scenery to add interest to their lives.

With the dog's advancing years, it is a good plan to begin to establish a routine walk that can be shortened if necessary. Thus, as the legs and sight begin to fail, the old dog is able to use his other senses to feel familiar in his surroundings even if the distance travelled is not as great as previously. Remember too to turn back for home while the dog still has plenty of energy.

AVOIDING OBESITY

As the body ages, all bodily systems age with it. Thus, the heart and circulation are not as efficient, neither are the lungs or the locomotor system, especially the muscles and joints. With advancing age these systems should be able to support and transport a dog of the correct weight but may fail if the dog is grossly overweight. Hearts fail, but even more frequently ligaments snap under the increased weight, thus crippling the dog. Arthritic changes are much more painful and significant in the overweight dog. Surveys show that sixty per cent of our patients are overweight and it is not uncommon for us to be presented with a dog whose weight is 40kg (90lbs) despite a breed average of 27kg (60lbs) – a fifty per cent increase. To put this in perspective, a human whose normal weight should be 64kg (10 stone) would weigh 95kg (15 stone) and be grossly overweight. Thus, a Miniature Dachshund whose normal weight should be 4.5kg (10lbs) would weigh 7kg (15lbs). This difference of only 2.25kg (5lbs) sounds very small but it is the *percentage* increase which is important.

Slimming Diet

Obviously a dog of normal weight will approach old age with a greater likelihood of reaching it. It follows, therefore, that it is timely to diet your dog as he approaches old age if you have let his weight gradually increase throughout his life. A diet is not for ever. It is usually for a short sharp period of perhaps twelve weeks, after which the food intake can be increased *almost* to normal if the weight loss has been achieved.

The aim of such a diet is to reduce the calorie intake to about sixty per cent of normal, to encourage the conversion of body fat back into energy. A high-fibre diet should be fed so that the dog's appetite is

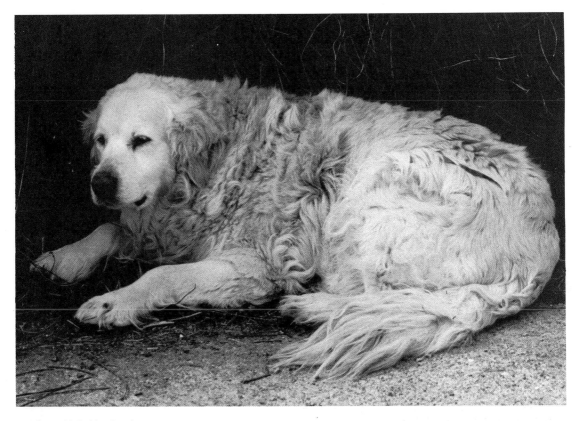

An obese old Golden Retriever.

satisfied and he does not feel hungry. Maintenance levels of essential nutrients such as protein, vitamins and minerals must be provided so that deficiencies do not occur.

Your veterinary surgeon will be able to advise on the choice of several prescription low calorie diets available in both dried and tinned form or you can mix your own to the following suggested formula.

Ingredients

115g (4oz) lean minced meat
75g (half cup) low fat cottage cheese
310g (2 cups) grated raw carrot
270g (2 cups) green runner beans
A balanced vitamin and mineral supplement (ask your vet for his recommendation)

Method

Cook the meat, pour away the fat and allow to cool. Add the remaining ingredients and mix thoroughly. Remember this is a complete diet and nothing else except water should be given to the dog until the weight loss has been achieved.

The diet should be fed at about the rate of 0.5kg food per 15kg body weight that the dog *should be*. To ensure that the dog remains healthy and loses weight, we would suggest a monthly visit to your vet to monitor progress.

EUTHANASIA

This is the medical term for the commonly used expression, 'putting to sleep'. Many will argue that vets and their patients have this advantage over the medical profession. Animals who are terminally ill, incurably in pain, or have lost essential body functions and have no chance of regaining a happy active life can have their life painlessly and peacefully ended.

The criteria for choosing euthanasia are fairly clear cut and it is very important for owners to understand that the vet can only euthanase their pets *with their consent*. All too commonly vets are presented with an old dog that they cannot help; the owner has left it too late because he was afraid to present the dog earlier in case the vet recommended euthanasia. No vet likes to lose a patient and where treatment is available it will be used. Conversely, the owner can override the vet's recommendation and request euthanasia for their dog. The vet has only two choices in this situation. He can either euthanase the dog as requested or politely refuse and refer the owner and patient away to another vet. We cannot, without the owner's consent, take the dog from the owner and find it a new home. With such consent, we can attempt to re-home young dogs which may be unsuitable for their particular owners.

Euthanasia is performed either for the benefit of the dog, or for the benefit of the owner or society in general.

Benefit of the Dog

The vast majority of euthanasias performed by vets are for the benefit of the dog. To assess the situation and decide whether euthanasia is necessary or not, the vet will consider the basic needs of a dog and whether they are being fulfilled. He will ascertain whether the dog has:

1 Freedom from pain, distress and discomfort. If not, can the pain be controlled?
2 The ability to walk and balance fairly well.
3 The ability to eat and drink without vomiting.
4 The freedom from inoperable tumours which are painful.
5 The ability to breathe without difficulty.
6 The ability to urinate and defaecate without difficulty or incontinence.
7 An owner who is able to cope physically and mentally with any nursing that may be needed.

If the answer to *any* of the above is no and treatment is not possible then the dog cannot live a normal happy life and euthanasia should be gently carried out.

Benefit of the Owner or Society in General

This category covers the dog which is a danger or a serious nuisance, where euthanasia is the only feasible answer. We are presented from time to time with dogs that, despite prolonged and serious attempts by owners to retrain them, have begun to bite people. No one should take the risk of a child being seriously harmed or killed by an aggressive dog. Dogs who worry sheep causing abortion or death may have a destruction order placed on them by a court of law. Euthanasia may have to be considered in dogs who habitually and irreversibly destroy their owner's furnishings and homes, attack every dog they see, or fail to become house-trained leading to both an aesthetic and a hygiene problem. Of course, dogs may have to be put to sleep in stray-dog homes just because there are too many dogs for too few good homes – the real answer to this is to prevent birth in the first place by neutering.

The Procedure

In the vast majority of cases, euthanasia is a smooth, peaceful transition from consciousness to unconsciousness, achieved by the injection into a front-leg vein of an overdose of an anaesthetic agent. This is the usual method employed by veterinary surgeons in most circumstances.

The dog is held in a sitting or lying position by a veterinary nurse or a competent owner and one foreleg is gently lifted at the elbow and held by this person. The paw so offered is held by the vet in his left hand while he carefully clips some hair from the dog's foreleg just below his elbow. Here runs a main vein, the cephalic vein, and it is into this that the injection is given. The vet will then usually apply surgical spirit to the skin to make the vein stand out while the nurse applies gentle pressure to the leg across the elbow to hold up the blood flow in the vein and make it possible for the vet to inject into it. This is called 'raising the vein'. The dog will be totally at ease as this position of sitting and giving a paw is one with which he is familiar and comfortable. If this procedure in any way upsets the dog or is made difficult by the dog for the vet, a sedative may be given first.

The vet inserts the needle painlessly into the vein and injects a concentrated solution of pentobarbitone - a triple-concentrated barbiturate anaesthetic prepared specially for this purpose. This is carried out in the vast majority of cases without the dog noticing; the speed of action is so rapid that unconsciousness ensues within five to ten seconds and the dog gently but quickly falls asleep on the table.

Within two minutes or so breathing ceases and shortly after this the heartbeat ceases. The transition is smooth and peaceful and there can be no kinder way of ending life when there is no alternative.

Coinciding with the cessation of the heartbeat and therefore the onset of death, there may be an odd shiver or twitch of a muscle or two. This is a nervous reflex and one that cannot be avoided. Occasionally if the nerves supplying the chest are involved, the dog may seem to take a breath. This is referred to as the 'last gasp' and can be a little disconcerting but of course the important thing is that the dog is totally unaware of this and at peace.

At Home or in the Surgery

In our opinion, an owner has the right to decide where euthanasia should take place. It is the last thing we will do for the patient and it should be carried out where it will cause the least distress for him. If the dog is sitting on the surgery table when the decision is reached, obviously it is not sensible to subject him to a further car journey or the owner to prolonged distress. If, however, the need is not immediate, when the time comes the owner should not have to transport an infirm old dog to the surgery if it would distress him. It should, however, be borne in mind that it may be easier for all concerned, and therefore better for the dog, if this is carried out in the surgery where expert help is readily available. A nurse, of course, can accompany the vet to the house if necessary.

To be Present or Not

This is again a decision for the individual owner. Some like to be present while others cannot entertain the idea. In general, unless the vet advises otherwise, we would recommend that you stay with your dog for the procedure rather than just leave him with the vet. The advantages are twofold: the dog is usually happier and calmer with the owner present and you, the owner, *know* exactly what happened and how peaceful it was.

233

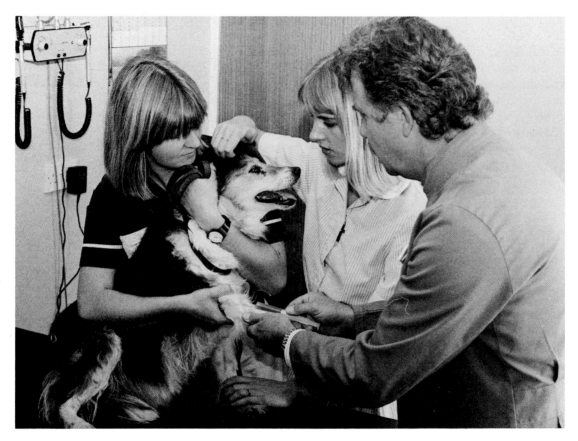

Euthanasia – a peaceful, caring solution when the time comes.

Disposal of the Body

Your vet will be able to advise you on the relative merits of the methods available to you depending on your locality. Cremation and burial are usually available and normally the vet will make the arrangements for you. Of course, you are at liberty to bury this important member of your family in your own garden. The important thing to remember is to bury him with at least two feet of soil over him and preferably in a cardboard or wooden box.

Afterwards

There are a few things you should, or should not, do. You have lost an old friend and, in most cases, a member of the family, so do allow yourself to grieve. It is completely normal and natural and you will feel better afterwards.

Do not reproach yourself for having taken his life – if the decision was a carefully considered one, on the vet's recommendation or with his agreement, you have made the correct choice. Do not blame yourself for losing the dog – death is rarely something that can be avoided by attention from the owner – and do not blame the vet for being unable to cure the dog of an incurable complaint!

Do not regard the death of your aged dog as a tragedy. It is not. It is very sad and you will miss him but death in old age is the most natural occurrence in the world.

Rather try and rejoice in his long life – you have lots of memories and reminders of him to help you.

Do not resist having another dog when the time comes, thinking it would be unfair on the old dog. It certainly would not – unless you are going to compare him with the new one. Dogs live ten to fifteen years, we live seventy to ninety years, so it is obvious we all may have many more than one dog during our lifetime. No dog ever replaces the one we lost, but they all have their own unique, lovable character.

There is a lot to be said for taking on a new puppy when your dog is approaching old age. This helps in two ways. Firstly, it will often give the old dog a new lease of life to have a playful companion, and, secondly, it helps you considerably during the grief period when the old dog eventually dies.

Index